EMERGENCY SERVICES
LEADERSHIP
A CONTEMPORARY APPROACH

David T. Foster, III, MLS, EMT-P

Brent J. Goertzen, PhD

Chris Nollette, EdD, NREMT-P, LP

Frank P. Nollette, MA, CMSGT, USAF (Retired)

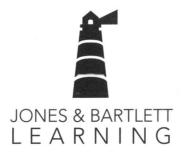

JONES & BARTLETT
LEARNING

World Headquarters
Jones & Bartlett Learning
5 Wall Street
Burlington, MA 01803
978-443-5000
info@jblearning.com
www.jblearning.com

Jones & Bartlett Learning books and products are available through most bookstores and online booksellers. To contact Jones & Bartlett Learning directly, call 800-832-0034, fax 978-443-8000, or visit our website, www.jblearning.com.

Substantial discounts on bulk quantities of Jones & Bartlett Learning publications are available to corporations, professional associations, and other qualified organizations. For details and specific discount information, contact the special sales department at Jones & Bartlett Learning via the above contact information or send an email to specialsales@jblearning.com.

Production Credits

Chairman, Board of Directors: Clayton Jones
Chief Executive Officer: Ty Field
President: James Homer
SVP, Editor-in-Chief: Michael Johnson
SVP, Chief Technology Officer: Dean Fossella
SVP, Chief Marketing Officer: Alison M. Pendergast
Executive Publisher: Kimberly Brophy
Vice President of Sales, Public Safety Group: Matthew Maniscalco
Director of Sales, Public Safety Group: Patricia Einstein
Executive Acquisitions Editor—EMS: Christine Emerton
Associate Production Editor: Nora Menzi
Director of Marketing: Alisha Weisman
V.P., Manufacturing and Inventory Control: Therese Connell

Composition: Abella Publishing Services
Cover Design: Kristin E. Parker
Rights and Permissions Manager: Katherine Crighton
Photo Research Supervisor: Anna Genoese
Permissions and Photo Research Assistant: Lian Bruno
Cover Images: Soldiers: Courtesy of Staff Sgt. Jacob N. Bailey/U.S. Air Force. Firemen at Scene of Accident: © Corbis. City skyline: © AbleStock, Fireman in protective helmet: © Jones & Bartlett Learning. Photographed by Glen E. Ellman. Police officer and cruiser: © Corbis. Two female officers at WTC site: Courtesy of Andrea Booher/FEMA.
Printing and Binding: Courier Kendallville
Cover Printing: Courier Kendallville

Library of Congress Cataloging-in-Publication Data
Emergency services leadership : a contemporary approach / David T. Foster III ... [et al.].
    p. ; cm.
  Includes bibliographical references and index.
  ISBN 978-0-7637-8150-7
  I. Foster, David T.
  [DNLM: 1. Emergency Medical Services. 2. Leadership. WX 215]
  LC-classification not assigned
  616.02'5—dc23
                    2011033475

6048
Printed in the United States of America
15 14 13 12 11   10 9 8 7 6 5 4 3 2 1

Contents

Acknowledgments

The authors and Jones & Bartlett Learning would like to thank the following reviewers for their expertise and guidance in the development of this text:

Brenda M. Beasley, RN, MS, EMT-P
Department Chair, Allied Health (Retired)
Calhoun Community College
Wedowee, Alabama

Bryan F. Ericson, MEd, RN, NREMT-P
Tarrant County College—EMS Program
Euless, Texas

David Loftin, BS, EMT-P
Georgia Office of EMS and Trauma–Region 1 (Retired)
Rome, Georgia

Phil G. Petty, BS, EMT-P
Technical College System of Georgia (retired)
Conyers, Georgia

Lisa Pitts, MLS, EMT
Hutchinson Community College
Washburn University
Hutchinson, Kansas

About the Authors

David T. Foster, III, MLS, EMT-P

Mr. David T. Foster's 36-year background in fire and emergency medical services (EMS) includes service in suppression, rescue, EMS, emergency preparedness, and training. His experience includes working in city, county, hospital-based, and federal installation response services. He also has regulatory and educational/training oversight experience with the Technical College System of Georgia as the EMS Programs Field Training Officer for Service Delivery Area 1 and later as the Region 1 Office of EMS as a Training Specialist. He is currently the Region 1 Program Director for the Georgia Office of EMS and Trauma. Over the past 10 years, Mr. Foster pursued an academic path to enhance his personal and professional knowledge. This journey led him to expand his teachings from the training room to the classroom. In recent years, he has been teaching leadership courses in the Department of Leadership at Fort Hays State University's Virtual College, where he teaches *Leadership and Team Dynamics* and *Introduction to Emergency Services Leadership* courses.

Brent J. Goertzen, PhD

Dr. Brent J. Goertzen has an extensive background in leadership theory and application. He holds a doctoral degree in community and human resources with a specialization in leadership studies from the University of Nebraska–Lincoln. Dr. Goertzen has more than 10 years of experience in teaching leadership coursework to undergraduate and graduate students, and he has done considerable work in the area of assessment of leadership education.

Chris Nollette, EdD, NREMT-P, LP

Dr. Chris Nollette rose through the fire service and EMS ranks. He has 30 years of experience and continues to be a leadership student, both as a researcher and as Program Director for Moreno Valley College, Riverside Community College District EMS Academy. Dr. Nollette is active in many national organizations, including the prestigious National Association of EMS Educators, where he most recently served as President. He is a founding member of the American Heart Association Scientific Subcommittee on Education and a past board member of the Committee for Accreditation of EMS

Paramedic Programs. He travels extensively on the conference circuits and speaks on leadership, mentoring, building people skills, emotional and social intelligence, and a variety of medical research topics.

Frank P. Nollette, MA, CMSGT, USAF (Retired)

Mr. Frank P. Nollette has an extensive military background. His specialty is in emergency preparedness and leadership training. His U.S. Air Force assignments include Aircrew Protection; Air Rescue; Special Operations; Nuclear, Biological, and Chemical Defense; and Disaster Control/Preparedness, including combat experience, Operational Planning, and Exercises in Southeast Asia. Throughout his military and civilian career in governmental human resources, he has taught, counseled, and mentored individuals, teams, and organizations. He has vast knowledge and experience in both the military and civilian applications of command and control and leadership development.

Preface

Ask a group of people to describe what leadership means and you will get many different answers. To some, leadership is about power or control. To others, it may describe the primary task of someone in a management position, such as an officer or supervisor. Still others may see it as the responsibility to build relationships among people working together. Our unique life experiences frame our individual perspectives on leadership.

The goal of this book is to expand your understanding of leadership—recognizing that, as your understanding of leadership grows, so will your capacity to lead. As you continue your journey through this text, you will begin to discover that many excellent commanders are poor leaders, and many good leaders are poor commanders. It is this balance of commanding and leading that we hope you, as a current or future leader, will come to appreciate and embrace.

We approach the subject of leadership from three directions: In Section 1, we delve into the past and take an historical look at the development of leadership concepts in the emergency service professions; Section 2 presents and explores the major leadership theories; and Section 3 offers real-world examples of leadership and allows the reader to see how history and theory are applied.

David T. Foster, III, MLS, EMT-P
Brent J. Goertzen, PhD
Chris Nollette, EdD, NREMT-P, LP
Frank P. Nollette, MA, CMSGT, USAF (Retired)

1

Leadership Past and Present

1

Introduction to Leadership

Chris Nollette and Frank P. Nollette

Winton Churchill faced an enormous dilemma before World War II. His fellow countrymen did not see the danger that lurked before them. He was criticized, and his reputation was questioned by his fellow countrymen. He stood alone in the face of an overwhelming feeling that Germany was no threat to the British Empire or the world; and yet, he knew the truth and his values, and his guiding principles urged him forward to sound the alarm on a sleeping empire at the edge of darkness.

▨ INTRODUCTION

All people have values, but the defining feature of moral courage is to have the courage to live according to one's values even in the face of tremendous pressure. Although most people struggle with doing what is right, a few do not hesitate; they move confidently forward, and their values are the guiding light and the principles that shape their lives. They put themselves in harm's way physically and emotionally, knowing that their very reputations and life are at risk in the face of enormous pressure to comply. These are the greatest heroes, for without them so many things would not have changed in this world, and so many wrongs would continue to prosper.

Since the beginning of time, leaders have evolved out of necessity to meet a critical need or ward off a terrible danger. There were no schools or textbooks that described what leadership was or should be; instead, an inner voice moved leaders forward. This moral courage is the very essence of leadership, and through time it has become a guiding force for many leaders. Winston Churchill understood the power of moral courage and how it could be a beacon to the masses during moments of crisis. It was a power that he would need to call on as his country was thrust into the depths of an epic struggle

for survival. Churchill, 65 years old and retired as Lord of the Admiralty and Prime Minister, was called back to service because of the force of his principles and the clarity of his values. On his first night back as Prime Minister at 10 Downing Street, with a whole nation turning to him for his moral leadership, Churchill wrote the following:

> *I was conscious of a profound sense of relief and I was inspired by a deep sense of destiny. I suddenly realized that all my past life had been but a preparation for this hour and for this trial.*

▨ EARLY MAN, EARLY LEADER

Where did the concept of leadership originate? Could early humans have thrived or even met their essential needs of food, water, and shelter without leaders? Theoretically, a small family group, clan, or tribe might have survived, or even prospered, under a communal model of social organization, given ideal conditions. However, outside influences that challenged a group's survival, such as the weather and changing seasons, threats from wild animals and other tribes, and the need to find food, would have required some response from the group to ensure its survival. Given what has been learned over years of study of the nature of humans, particularly in social interactions, consensus was probably very hard to achieve without efficient communication processes. Therefore, one can imagine that a group's survival would have been directly influenced by the presence of a leader who could pull everyone together to help achieve an optimum response to external threats.

It is likely that these early leaders emerged by virtue of being the strongest physically, the most intelligent, or the most successful hunters. Because early humans led a nomadic existence, the more successful hunter-gatherers likely would have attracted a following among the other families or tribal members. Individuals who could provide a steady supply of food would understandably be looked on with some form of admiration or respect, if for no other reason than to ensure that followers could share in the bounty of the hunt. From this position of strength, such individuals could wield enormous influence over their groups. In addition, skills that directly enhanced survival, such as foraging for edible plants, preserving food, and medicinal knowledge, may also have given rise to leadership roles, along with status-enhancing elements, such as knowledge of tribal lore and shamanic traditions.

As villages, towns, and cities developed over the millennia, additional specialization became essential to cooperative and communal living. Planting and harvesting of grain and related crops, the domestication and breeding of animals, the development of religions, and a burgeoning understanding of the physical world about them required new expertise. Physical and later military prowess was also required of many to ensure the safety and well-being of the locale and peoples, at first in defensive roles (which led to the building of barriers and walls, and later cities, to protect the citizens and stores of food, which were of great interest to the still-nomadic tribes) and most likely in internal policing of the group. Crop failures, natural disasters, war, or other events may have depleted the resources of the group, leading its citizens to seek the resources of other groups in nearby or even distant lands. Groups capable of such conquests, whether well-organized warrior classes or simply bands of stronger individuals capable of waging warfare on an ad hoc basis, would have required some form of effective leadership. By consensus, or perhaps by brute force, there likely would have emerged a "leader of leaders" with more sweeping powers, or perhaps one who had the

diplomatic skills to hold together a loose confederation within the village, town, or city.

A great deal of effort and skill was required to convince strong warriors that, although the pursuit of them was dangerous, desired objectives were attainable and victory would be theirs with cooperation. The same is true today as militaries, naval forces, and emergency services orchestrate effective, collective responses to potentially hazardous situations. Firefighters often say in jest, illustrating the immense difficulty of this challenge, "Why is it that when a structure is ablaze, the rats and even the cockroaches evacuate the area while firefighters rush in?" Why do police officers run toward gunfire and noise while civilians run in the other direction? Why do emergency medical technicians and paramedics place themselves at risk to tend to victims? How do members of the military overcome the very human desire to flee rather than fight when they know that they risk injury and even death when going into battle? The natural reaction that humans experience when faced with peril must be suppressed in the warrior (this includes firefighters, police officers, and emergency medical services [EMS] providers) in favor of loyalty to one's fellow warriors, to one's leaders, to one's mission or objectives, and perhaps foremost to one's self. In such situations, the police and fire chief, the EMS director, and emergency management officials are like military commanders, wrestling constantly with the dilemma of how to use their resources with minimal risk and the least likelihood of injury or death to responders while accomplishing their essential goals.

ARE LEADERS BORN OR MADE?

One school of thought maintains that certain individuals have innate talents, will, and predisposition to become leaders. It is held that the destiny of such individuals is to rise to positions of leadership in whatever field they find themselves. Examples are often cited where leaders were born into nobility or royalty and achieved great things as they took their expected and exalted positions. Other writers extol the virtues of notable leaders of more humble birth who exhibited at an early age some or many of the talents and qualities expected of a leader. These "born leaders" can be found throughout history, and there is no doubt that some individuals seem to be destined for greatness from an early age.

However, in all likelihood, the formative years of any great leader include intense education, training, and ideally practical experience in the arts of governance and leadership. One well-known contemporary example of this is the British monarchy. Princes William and Harry, heirs apparent to the British crown, have scarcely been languishing about Windsor Castle or Buckingham Palace, awaiting their dates with destiny. Both have been well schooled in their roles as leaders. They were educated at Eton, serve in the British armed forces, and represent their Queen and country abroad on diplomatic and humanitarian missions.

Similarly, one can trace many of America's great industrial and commercial leaders, such as the Rockefellers, Du Ponts, and Carnegies, through their bloodlines. In virtually all instances, however, members of these prominent families likewise underwent schooling, training, and perhaps even mentorship in preparation for the roles into which they were born. In cases where an individual lacks adequate preparation and credentials and ascends to a leadership position solely through birthright, vested authority eventually gives way, as the individual becomes a figurehead rather than a true leader.

One other important factor in the development of great leaders, whether or not they were born into their positions, is opportunity. For the purpose of this book, opportunity is defined as the chance to demonstrate leadership abilities. In the field of public safety, opportunity comes each time one is summoned to respond to a call for help. These opportunities allow one to define their own bit of greatness as they handle the stress and complexity that all leaders face during critical times. These moments come in short and wild bursts but are no less significant than the moments or opportunities faced by great political and military leaders. One only has to think of Winston Churchill, who stood alone in the House of Commons during World War II as he stated, "I am your servant. You have the right to dismiss me when you please. What you have no right to do is ask me to bear responsibility without the power of action." Winston Churchill seized his opportunity, rose to greatness, and saved a nation in the process.

Another school of thought holds that virtually everyone, regardless of genetics or birthright, has the potential to become a leader and needs only adequate education, training, and preparation. Napoleon Bonaparte once said (roughly translated) that in every private's knapsack is a

marshal's baton, alluding to the fact that even the lowliest of soldiers might someday, at some time and place, exhibit the leadership qualities expected of a Marshal of France. In the throes of accidents, disasters, and war, some individuals suddenly rise to leadership for relatively brief moments, leading their comrades or even strangers through or out of danger. The authors have seen these "sudden leaders" emerge in dangerous situations, man-made and natural disasters, accidents, and combat. In the chaos of the situation, and in the absence of more easily identified or designated leadership, it takes but one individual to raise his or her voice to galvanize others into action. Even not knowing if the voice emanates from one trained or designated as a leader, a group at risk gravitates toward such an individual, because guidance of any kind offers some semblance of hope when one feels overwhelmed by the situation. The emergency services community trains for emergencies, disasters, and perils. Military and naval forces train for such situations, but they train even more intensely for operations amid the chaos and confusion of warfare. By virtue of training, experience, and personal character, individuals in each of these realms, civilian and military, have the potential to become leaders, even for brief periods.

The events of September 11, 2001, particularly in New York City, spotlighted the hundreds of untrained civilians who suddenly became leaders and took action to cope with the disaster unfolding around them. They led others to stairwells, sent people to safety at the risk of their own, urged others to help one another, and in countless other ways saved many lives. This in no way denigrates the efforts of the professional and volunteer firefighters, police officers, and EMS workers, all of whom had the advantage of training and experience to help them cope with the essentials (although hardly the magnitude) of the situations they were facing. Maybe Napoleon was correct when he thought that a leader lurks in everyone, and a given situation could bring leadership to the forefront.

Take a moment and think of the last time you had an opportunity to take a leadership role. Maybe it was during a critical call, maybe it was helping to mentor a new recruit, or maybe it was as simple as seizing a teachable moment with one of your kids. Opportunities to step up and demonstrate leadership come every day. Unfortunately, many times people let opportunity pass by and, in doing so, lose the chance to help themselves and others grow, for as one lifts up those around them, one also rises in the process.

> ## Leadership Points to Ponder
>
> *Leaders aren't born, they are made. And they are made just like anything else, through hard work. And that's the price we'll have to pay to achieve that goal, or any goal.*
>
> Vince Lombardi (from *http://thinkexist.com*)

THE LEADER IN ALL OF US

One of the greatest propaganda coups of World War II fostered by the Allied Powers was the notion that common enemy soldiers and sailors were unable to function when they lost their leaders. Supposedly, the loss of a unit commander or other leader would leave the troops in confusion, unsure of what to do next. The belief was that these troops would easily fall prey to the more motivated and better-led American forces. Reality proved otherwise in many instances, much to the surprise of the Americans and their allies, when other individuals stepped up to take on a leadership role.

War histories are replete with tales of how individual soldiers, sailors, and airmen rose to sudden prominence in the heat of battle or major adversity, assuming the heavy burden of leadership under the most trying circumstances. Although there are many contemporary examples one can point to in the public safety professions, one only has to look at what occurred on that fateful day in New York City on September 11, 2001, in the World Trade Towers, where the command structure was taken out when the second tower came down. Although this event had the opportunity to cripple the response, new leaders stepped up and, in their darkest hour, took over and kept the response moving forward, saving many lives that otherwise could have been lost.

Public safety professionals have to take on a leadership role each and every day. EMS, fire, and law enforcement have had to create layers of leadership to be able to control scenes and work mass casualty events to take care of the sick and injured. Everyone must be able to fill gaps as needed; survival demands that people work together so that the patient and the rescuer have a positive outcome. Leadership lies in each person, and cultivating leadership must be a priority for any organization.

Being Prepared When Opportunity Knocks

Opportunities for leadership abound, even in day-to-day lives, but if one is unprepared for leadership, the opportunities will pass them by. This textbook is intended to aid in the preparation for the time when the opportunity to exercise leadership presents itself. Ask yourself the following questions:

- What can I offer to this position and to the mission at hand?
- Where are my talents and where are my deficiencies?
- How many mentors should I have to accomplish the task at hand?
- Am I a team player?
- Is my attitude a positive one?
- Am I a person of influence?
- Do I have a courageous heart to know my limitations and understand that people are more important than process?

These are just a few of the questions one must explore in oneself and with the people one leads. Too often leaders are caught up in the mystique of leadership and not focused on the substance of leadership.

> ## Leadership Points to Ponder
>
> *Being powerful is like being a lady. If you have to tell people you are, you aren't.*
>
> Former British Prime Minister, Margaret Thatcher (from *http://thinkexist.com*)

LEADER OR MANAGER

One must clearly define and contrast the definitions of a leader and a manager. Although many of the essential qualities are the same or similar for both roles, there are distinct differences. Managers focus on maintaining systems related to day-to-day operations, whereas leaders are those who can influence people, see beyond process to the big picture, and bring different perspectives to problem solving. Most importantly, leaders take responsibility for developing their followers and helping them reach their fullest potential. Leaders can create change in positive and productive ways, a critical skill in a changing and dynamic environment. This is not to say that managers are not important; a good manager must deftly handle the responsibilities of task, time, process control, personnel assignments, and the many other duties that require managing. Many of the officers in emergency services are excellent managers, on and off the emergent scene. It is clear, however, that managers and leaders serve two different roles.

MORAL LEADERSHIP

The notion of "moral leadership" is also important to the overall question of what makes a leader. Moral leadership is not reserved for members of the clergy in guiding their flocks through moral dilemmas. Opportunities present themselves daily for leaders to display a sense of morality. A leader, whether exercising leadership by virtue of positional authority or having unconsciously assumed the role of leader by his or her actions, exercises moral leadership by adherence to a personal code of ethics that merits emulation by peers, subordinates, and even superiors.

In the 1950s, the U.S. military decided that moral leadership was so critical that it implemented training for all ranks in this subject. During the late 1950s and early 1960s, the U.S. Air Force required unit commanders to provide moral leadership training and lectures to all personnel. The content of most of these lectures focused on the need for individuals to conduct themselves, whether on or off duty, in a manner consistent with contemporary morals and the unique demands of military service as spelled out in rules, regulations, the Code of Conduct (for those captured), the Universal Code of Military Justice, and the Geneva Conventions (e.g., Laws of Land/Air Warfare; Rules of Engagement; Treatment of Civilians, Enemies, POWs). Ethics and morals training has become an essential and practical part of building good leaders and has been integrated throughout all of the armed services, beginning in basic training and continuing through the mandatory training and education of both enlisted and officer corps.

Leadership Points to Ponder

There is a secret pride in every human heart that revolts at tyranny. You may order and drive an individual, but you cannot make him respect you.

William Hazlitt (from *http://quotationsbook.com*)

For too long, the public safety professions of EMS, fire, and police have approached moral leadership as a side topic—a seminar talk—and have failed to see this as

critical to the mission of public safety. More time is spent on legal issues and how to protect the individual and the service from getting into trouble, whether through bad press or financial liability, when the real focus should be on developing leaders with a moral compass.

Many leaders do not understand the difference between values and ethics. Values can be described as inner judgments or beliefs that guide one through life's trials and tribulations in both professional and personal settings. Values develop over time and are shaped by one's environment. If a leader values family, it could be rooted in the fact that they never really had a family of their own, they came from a great family that they want to reproduce for themselves, or their experiences were not positive and they want the chance to experience the real meaning of a family. Whatever the reason, an inner voice drives this value forward and it becomes an intrinsic value that may come in conflict with their work ethics. Others have the value of family but do not allow that value to be a driving force in their lives. They say family is important to them but work a tremendous amount of overtime with the belief that providing more things will secure them to their family. The national divorce rate speaks well to this subject when so many lose sight of their value and in turn lose what they believed at one time was a guiding principle of their lives. Values must be a part of a leader's tool bag but those tools must be well worn with use or they simply become confusing and unused. Leaders must reflect on what values they embrace, because only through an understanding of these values can real, meaningful change occur.

Ethics has been described as "good or right behavior accepted by society"; if distilled into just one word, ethics can be thought of as "behavior." Ethics differs from values, and they are clearly two different words that must be thought of as distinct and separate. Values (beliefs) drive ethics (behavior). When leaders understand their values for better or worse, then they begin to understand why they behave the way they do in given situations. The problem is that so many in society do not understand or have not even reflected on their values. When one does not understand their values, it is impossible to really understand or change their behavior. It is critical that every profession have a foundation of ethical guidelines. Unfortunately, any code of ethics, which is nothing more than a list of things "thou profession and professionals shall not do," has come about because someone did the wrong thing. Only through an unwavering commitment to the highest standards of professionalism can one hope to protect the ideals that they have sworn to uphold. In the book *Making Ethical Decisions* (Josephson, 2002), there is mention of the six pillars of character: (1) trustworthiness, (2) respect, (3) responsibility, (4) fairness, (5) caring, and (6) citizenship. Perhaps these can be the guiding force for leaders because they are universal concepts that everyone may agree on as essential, foundational pieces for emerging and current leaders. Having a moral compass is not only for leaders but also for all members of an organization, who must follow the right path and keep moving in the right direction.

MENTORING FOR LEADERSHIP

Researchers have long stressed how important mentoring is from a professional standpoint. It is a critical component of leadership in any field, and none more so than the field of public safety, where the lives and well-being of the public and the professionals who serve them are at stake. It is more critical today than it was in the past, because the world is much more complicated and there is constant change to professional landscapes.

All professionals have a duty to share their wisdom, their purpose, and their passion with the next generation. Doing so inspires others and perhaps helps them find their calling to serve, thereby growing the field in a positive and purposeful manner. Although mentoring is really defined as a long-term relationship, it can span a lifetime or simply be a moment in time. Many are fearful of asking for help, because they believe it will show them to be less capable and intelligent. No one can have all the answers; people must depend on each other for support.

Vision is the foundation for mentoring, because it is through true vision that a person sees the world not as what it is but what it can become. People realize the mistakes they have made or the opportunities they have missed and want the next generation to do better. A great mentor helps others to realize the greatness in themselves. Mother Teresa, Cesar Chavez, Martin Luther King, and Gandhi were great mentors of their generations. Their visions galvanized people around the globe to address pressing, large-scale social issues and, in the process, rekindled the human spirit. Where others saw a present replete with problems, they saw a future of great possibilities and worked tirelessly to realize that vision. In an abstract sense, they mentored a whole generation to believe that the world can have greater justice.

The work of leaders and mentors in emergency services may not have the same global reach. Time may be spent in one district, working on one special training initiative, or helping that one young recruit who needs encouragement. The important thing is that, as leaders, they always strive to help others grow and fulfill their potential. The hope is to make the current generation, and the ones that follow, proud.

Leadership Points to Ponder

When the competitive nature overtakes the cooperative approach, there are winner and losers.

But even winners lose if they lose the trust and respect of their competitors.

CONCLUSION

There is no one strategy or miracle method that makes good or great leaders. The secret is to create and encourage an environment where failures can be accepted and even embraced as long as one "fails forward" and learning occurs. This type of learning leads to growth, and this becomes the one saving grace of all leaders: the ability to grow and learn from one's mistakes.

Leadership is based in theory, but the conversation is incomplete if there is no thought in the application of this theory. When leadership is applied, one begins to breathe life into and bring clarity to a complex subject. The authors' intent for this text is to blend the science of leadership (theory) with the art of leadership, otherwise known as the "humanistic qualities" (application). When these two areas come together, a servant leader begins to take shape and the true effectiveness of leadership begins to occur.

Leadership Points to Ponder

One day when Gandhi was on a train pulling away from the station, a European reporter running alongside his compartment continued to beg him to give him a message to take back to his readers concerning his life. It was a day of silence for Gandhi, part of his regular practice, so he did not reply. Instead, he scribbled a few words on a piece of paper and passed it to the journalist: "My life is my message." Just as Gandhi embraced a cause that defined his life, so must each person find a cause and each day build a message and a legacy, not on words but on deeds. This is the kind of message that will live on in the hearts and minds of those who follow, so that one's bit of greatness outlives their brief time on earth.

Wrap-Up

ACTIVITY

Ask those who care about you to assist you in assessing your strengths and weaknesses as a person. It is akin to holding up a mirror to yourself, one that knows you and can talk back.

Step 1: Create a list of your strengths and weaknesses. Bullet points will do. For example:

- Strengths
  - Honest
  - Funny
  - Disciplined
- Weaknesses
  - Short-tempered
  - Impatient

Step 2: Have loved ones look at your list and give their input. Perhaps you think you are funny, but a loved one disagrees and says you are sarcastic (a common weakness among military and public safety professionals).

Step 3: Once you have completed your list, develop a plan for improving on your weaknesses and enhancing your strengths.

REFERENCE

Josephson, M. (2002). *Making ethical decisions: The six pillars of character*. Los Angeles, CA: Josephson Institute of Ethics.

CHAPTER

Historical Perspectives

David T. Foster III and Frank P. Nollette

One day in 1832, while marching a couple dozen men across a field, a leader found an obstacle in his way: a fence with a narrow opening stood in his company's path. The leader guiding these men could not think of a command to get his men from one side to the other. Recounting the incident later in life, he said, "I could not for the life of me remember the proper word of command for getting my company endwise. Finally, as we came near (the gate) I shouted: This company is dismissed for two minutes, when it will fall in again on the other side of the gate." This leader went from captain to a private during the Black Hawk Wars and found that on reaching the lower rank, he performed at an acceptable level. The leader was Abraham Lincoln.

INTRODUCTION

This chapter addresses the development of the more comprehensive command and control and incident management models in widespread use today in the emergency services (ES) community and the critical contribution of the military to these systems. Although seldom appreciated or even recognized, the current ES community's processes, procedures, organizations, and management are rooted in military history. In today's world, the ES has developed even closer ties with state and federal military agencies. ES agencies (fire, police, emergency medical services [EMS], and emergency planners and managers) are organized, led, and managed primarily along paramilitary lines with distinct differences from the military in terms of expectations of individual performances. The military model provides a viable working structure, a well-defined chain of command, and a system of rules, regulations, and standards—all of which contribute to the cohesiveness of any ES program.

Not unlike the military, most ES community leaders have ascended to positions of greater responsibility through experience, training, personal initiative, and competitive processes. There are designated, appointed, volunteer, or elected officials who oversee or may directly or indirectly manage ES programs, but there are parallels in military history and in the present day, with a civilian in charge (the president, as commander in chief) down through the various civilian secretaries at various levels. At the state level, the governor has responsibilities for emergency and contingency planning, typically delegated to the respective state national guard agencies, which again reinforces the military organizational, operational, and management elements that can readily be adopted by the civilian community.

This chapter explores Firefighting Resources of California Organized for Potential Emergencies (FIRESCOPE) and the Incident Command System (ICS), developed in California in the 1970s, and how ICS eventually came to form the backbone of the current National Incident Management System (NIMS) approach at the federal level. The chapter concludes with a discussion of the collaboration between the military and civilian organizations. A careful assessment of how teamwork can solve problems has taken leadership to new levels. Never before have the military and public safety entities worked so closely to mitigate and respond to natural and man-made threats. This is the paradigm of the future for leadership.

FIRESCOPE

In 1970, several major wildfires ravaged the chaparral region of southern California. During a 13-day period, 16 lives were lost, more than half a million acres were burned, and more than 700 structures were destroyed (Irwin, 1981). The lessons learned during this tragic event led to the formation of FIRESCOPE, made up of several forestry, fire, and ES agencies at the federal, state, county, and municipal levels. Responders faced a number of challenges in battling the California blazes, including:

- Terminology differed from one agency to another: Each agency had a variety of terms for the same equipment, resulting in considerable confusion.

- Management of responders was hampered by the inability to expand and contract as needed: There were no distinct plans for how commanders would deploy units and resources when needed or how to stand them down when they were not needed.

- Response plans of different agencies were inconsistent: As with terminology, each agency had its own way of doing things, resulting in a lack of consistency and sometimes even leading to fights over who should do a particular task or how it should be done.

- Common communication channels did not exist: Each agency had its own radio frequencies. There were no common channels that all responders could use. This led to delays in the spread of information and increased confusion.

In 1971, Congress approved funding for research, led by FIRESCOPE technical teams, that was designed to improve fire command and control systems. This in turn led to the research program at the Pacific Southwest Forest and Range Experiment Station's Forest Fire Laboratory in Riverside, California. Members of the research team soon concluded that no patchwork of incremental improvements would suffice and that large, systemic changes were needed:

> This analysis quickly showed that the solution must involve a major systems design that would necessarily address not only advanced airborne fire

intelligence methods, but fire information systems generally and their effective utilization in planning and coordinating action on both single- and multiple-agency fires or similar emergencies. (Chase, 1980)

According to the Federal Emergency Management Agency's (FEMA) history of FIRESCOPE, two major innovations came out of this work: ICS and the Multi-Agency Coordination System (MACS). FEMA goes on to describe the effectiveness and significance of ICS:

> The first was that the ICS became widely used by the majority of fire service agencies in southern California as early as 1981 and then spread through the fire service across the country. The second was that the ICS was suitable for use in responses other than just fire fighting—to manage incidents such as natural disasters, major crashes, hazardous materials, and even large-scale public gatherings.

As the project moved into the early 1980s, fire departments across the country began adopting ICS. FIRESCOPE developed an ICS training course that was being taught and modified around the country to help fireground commanders operate more effectively and efficiently during all types of incidents. Many federal agencies also adopted the operational processes of ICS, culminating with the inclusion of ICS as a central component of NIMS.

MACS AND UNIFIED COMMAND

MACS, a process designed to manage large-scale responses that require greater resources and information management, was developed out of the FIRESCOPE partnership. The main roles of MACS are to support collaborative incident management, facilitate logistics and resources, coordinate information specific to the incident, and coordinate interagency and intergovernmental issues. MACS builds on the concept of unified command (UC). UC is a consensus-based, multiagency approach to scene management, where each agency has some responsibility for the incident and agency representatives work together to make decisions. No single agency takes the lead, because this approach would violate the core principles of UC:

> Although several organizations have attempted to introduce the concept of Lead Agency into UC, it can

prove ineffective, especially during the early phases. The concurrent nature of the strategic objectives would essentially require that the lead agency change from moment to moment. (Walsh et al., 2005)

As can be seen from this statement, it is extremely difficult for a single person or agency to manage incidents by themselves. Effective UC representatives need a leadership foundation that is based on relationships, ethics, service, transformation, and other theories of leadership equally with their ability to manage tasks and personnel.

ICS

ICS brought to the ES fields a standardized approach to incident management and incorporated the following key improvements over prior approaches: a common set of terms, procedures, and processes; a revised organizational structure; improved communications; and updated data collection and analysis systems. ICS gives fire, EMS, law enforcement, and other agencies a standardized approach to managing both large-scale and smaller, everyday incidents. ICS is based on command and control. In this model, leadership is considered a position, and each position has direct authority to manage and lead its respective sectors. There are five major components of the original ICS model: (1) incident command position, (2) planning, (3) operations, (4) logistics, and (5) finance and administration. A sixth component that may be included is information and intelligence. This component would be used primarily in law enforcement operations where there is a suspicion of a crime being committed. It could also be used in a military operation to gather intelligence about the enemy.

During most responses, the incident commander is the sole person in charge of scene management. However, in large-scale incidents that require a multiagency response, other leadership roles come into play. Initially, the incident commander is the highest-ranking person of the first units to arrive on the scene. If the first person on the scene is a junior-level police officer or paramedic, for example, he or she is the initial incident commander. As more units arrive, the highest-ranking officer within each agency assumes command on arrival. In large-scale, multiagency responses, this can be confusing unless the area jurisdiction set up a common incident command person for the incident. Too often, the authors have seen

law enforcement, EMS, and fire respond to a motor vehicle crash where the ranking fire or police office declares himself or herself the commander, when the incident is really a medical incident until patients are removed from the scene. A jurisdictional agreement whereby during medical calls the EMS officer is the commander, crime scenes have law enforcement in charge, and fire scenes have fire officers in charge would improve these responses immensely.

FIREGROUND COMMAND

As ICS was being developed and implemented, another model of command and control was also being developed in the fire service. Chief Alan V. Brunacini of the Phoenix Fire Department in Arizona, who was penning his renowned text *Fire Command*, was truly a leader, not only in his city, but also nationally and internationally. He was a visionary who realized that the fire service needed a systematic approach to fireground command. Where FIRESCOPE was designed to primarily address wildland fire command and the issues of multiagency responses, Chief Brunacini's system was designed to address the everyday response by individual fire departments and their operations not requiring multiagency response, and it became the norm for many fire departments throughout the United States in the 1980s. Many of Chief Brunacini's concepts seemed to parallel the ICS model already in place, yet were refined to be specific to structural and rescue operations of the fire service with a single incident commander:

An effective fireground operation centers around one incident commander. If there is no command, or if there are multiple commands, fireground operations quickly break down in seven predictable areas:

- *Action*
- *Command and control*
- *Coordination*
- *Planning*
- *Organization*
- *Communications*
- *Safety*

(Brunacini, 1985)

Chief Brunacini's vision was that the fireground commander is responsible not only for the management of the scene, but also for the safety and survival of the firefighters operating on scene. A commander's tasks include, but are not limited to, the protection, removal, and care of endangered occupants; stopping the fire; and conservation of property during and after the operation. Ultimately, fireground commanders are "expected to manage risks, develop effective communications, develop effective organizations and eliminate confusion" (Brunacini, 1985, p. 5). Successful fireground commanders are well versed in what Chief Brunacini called "selective democracy," meaning that they know when to collaborate with other on-scene personnel by taking a vote and when not to, always being aware that they hold the responsibility and authority to make definitive decisions. Fireground command is not really about an almighty scene dictator; it is about one person who is held accountable for the successful execution of the operational plan. Stephen Covey refers to the importance of execution in his book *The 8th Habit* (2004). Covey says that he would prefer to have excellent execution of a mediocre plan than a great plan and poor execution. When there is no coordination at the scene, multiple commanders create confusion by giving conflicting orders to responders; units operate independently, creating potentially unsafe and duplicated actions; and aspects of the scene can be ignored, resulting in poor outcomes.

In his text, Chief Brunacini breaks down all aspects of scene management. The first arriving unit establishes commanded. Once a high-ranking officer arrives, command is passed off to that officer, along with a full report of all actions and results before this point. This concept is now common practice in all ES sectors. First arriving crews establish command and control. The commander initially may be directly involved with response tasks and scene management. The following scenario illustrates the approach.

Operators from a 911 center dispatch three ambulances, two engine companies, one rescue squad, and several police officers to a multivehicle crash. Medic 4 arrives first with an emergency medical technician and a paramedic. The medic establishes command and begins to assess the scene. He or she makes decisions based on initial findings and may begin to triage patients while giving instructions to responding units. The EMS supervisor, an engine company, and two police officers arrive at the same time. Command is passed to the EMS supervisor, who then establishes a fixed command post and, collectively with the fire officer and senior police officer,

establishes such sectors as staging, extrication, transport, and traffic control. Local protocol calls for EMS to be in charge until all patients are removed; however, the commander realizes that he needs tremendous support from law enforcement and fire, so he coordinates with the senior officers of these agencies to manage the scene. Once all patients are treated and transported, command is passed from the EMS supervisor to the ranking fire officer for cleanup and resolution. Once all aspects of the fire service functions are completed, command is passed to the ranking police officer, who continues to manage the traffic and investigative segment of the operation to termination. The same concepts Chief Brunacini applied to fireground command are applied today to all response agencies.

NIMS

Expanding on ICS, FIRESCOPE, Fireground Command, and other similar approaches to scene management, NIMS evolved as a true national standard to be used in incident management and coordination:

> All events require effective and efficient coordination either within a single organization or across the broad spectrum of organizations and activities. The NIMS establishes a systems approach to integrate the most effective of existing processes and methods into a unified national framework for incident management. (Walsh et al., 2005)

NIMS originated in the Homeland Security Presidential Directive 5 of February 28, 2003. NIMS is a systematic, all-encompassing approach to managing every aspect of incident response from inception to termination, and it provides a consistent terminology to be used by all responders. NIMS has changed incident management from mainly task management to a process of collaboration. NIMS is not limited to the public safety sector. Other stakeholders can make use of the framework, such as public works; public health; local, state, and federal government agencies; volunteer agencies; and business partners.

MILITARY HISTORY OF ICS AND NIMS

The armed services have developed and published various contingency plans and detailed technical guidance to cope with natural disasters and man-made threats to readiness and resources. These plans contributed substantially to the development of ICS and NIMS. Military contingency plans address the ultimate disaster—that of warfare—but for events other than war, there is an entire host of potential threats to the military's readiness. The principles of planning for a natural or man-made disaster mimic those of planning for war, and most of the emergency service communities have used such precedents to develop their own plans and programs. Indeed, if one looks at the people who devised previous civilian programs, such as ICS, one finds a number of individuals with direct military experience in the planning, training, and exercising of contingency operations.

A review of much of the current preparedness literature, plans, and procedures shows an indelible Air Force stamp. Air Force Manual 355-1—a core documentation of responsibilities, standards, processes, and procedures—provided the first comprehensive, service-wide program to address disaster control (later changed to disaster preparedness) for all echelons of command and organization. The manual included direction on the planning and execution of unclassified postattack actions, such as development and management of fallout and chemical shelters. The various major air commands (such as what was then called Strategic Air Command, Tactical Air Command, Air Training Command, and others) tailored the programs to their own unique needs, but all had as their underlying core the U.S. Air Force guidance. Today, this guidance can be found in two extensive Air Force publications: Air Force Policy Directive 10-25, *Emergency Management* (U.S. Air Force, 2007), and Air Force Instruction (AFI) 10-2501, *Air Force Emergency Management Program* (U.S. Air Force, 2010). These same directives apply to the Air Force Reserve and Air National Guard forces and installations. Given that many statewide emergency preparedness organizations are typically assigned within the National Guard's headquarters elements, it is no wonder that the Air Force's programs are frequently mirrored to some degree in state policies and procedures.

The Navy had perhaps the nearest corollary to the Air Force's comprehensive program, but this was primarily centered on individual ships and other vessels. Aboard a ship or any other vessel, no matter the size, comprehensive plans, programs, and procedures (and the associated training and exercises) are essential for dealing with virtually any contingency. What the authors learned (to their astonishment) was that as late as 1980, there was no comprehensive Navy-level program for shore-based facilities, such as the Air Force program. Although each shore facility had various fire bills and emergency bills for some contingencies, most were left to their own devices in terms of an installation-wide response when there were two or more commands or agencies operating on the same site. Mutual aid agreements between agencies on Navy bases were in force for critical elements (e.g., fire and rescue, medical, security) but lacked the comprehensive programs that marked the Air Force's approach to preparedness.

All services and their installations have had their own fire departments, law enforcement agencies, medical providers, and command and control staffs, but disaster preparedness as a comprehensive program was fragmented. Subject matter experts and specialists, such as the Army's chemical-biological-radiological group, could cope with some aspects of preparedness and response. Navy radiological safety or reactor specialists are well versed in dealing with radiological incidents, but as in the Army chemical-biological-radiological community, there was a lack of comprehensive planning, command and control, mitigation, and recovery from major incidents at the installation level. The Air Force was the first service to have officer, enlisted, and civilian personnel assigned to a primary duty of disaster preparedness. By assigning a small cadre of technically qualified disaster preparedness personnel to each installation (staffing typically based on peak base population), the Air Force was able to create a comprehensive, service-wide program that complemented other contingency plans and operations at relatively minor cost. All the services now have personnel assigned to disaster preparedness, emergency management, or similar functional areas in recognition of the need for adequate program sustenance. Many of these personnel, on retirement or early separation, took those planning and training skills into the civilian realm and became valued contributors to virtually all state and local emergency plans and programs. If one compares the early California plans to the then-current AFM 355-1, one sees startling parallels or even direct excerpts from the manual for many of the specific procedures, organizations, communications, and training, including the development, execution, and assessment of exercises. **Figure 2-1** and **Table 2-1**, both from AFI 10-2501, show the

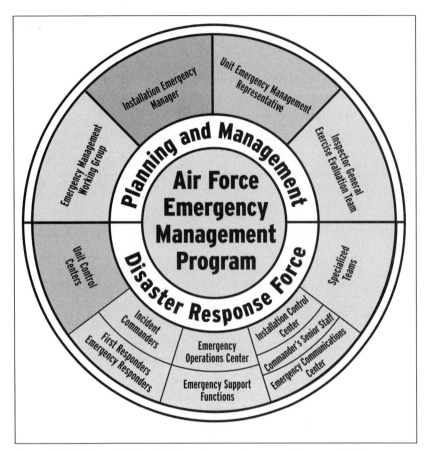

Source: U.S. Air Force. (2010). Air Force emergency management program. Air Force Instruction 10-2501, p. 23.

Figure 2-1 Air Force Emergency Management Program.

components of the Air Force Emergency Management programs and how they are mirrored or replicated in other systems of preparedness and response, particularly in NIMS.

In the early era of disaster preparedness development (especially in the years after the Vietnam War), military planning specialists had to convince commanders at all levels, from the smallest detachment or flight leaders up through Major Command Headquarters staff, that disaster preparedness was not a stand-alone function or just something requiring an annual exercise for record-keeping purposes. Senior disaster preparedness officers and noncommissioned officers emphasized at every opportunity that disaster preparedness is an integral part of management and leadership. Contingency plans, and even day-to-day operations, require consideration and planning for worst-case scenarios. Failure to plan for (or to practice) emergency procedures represents a significant flaw in management and leadership.

In the civilian world, disaster preparedness, by whatever name, is likewise an essential element of effective planning and preparation for the wide spectrum of both natural and manmade threats now faced. When local governments had to fund essential ES out of their own austere budgets, comprehensive emergency preparedness was often in the "nice to have" category and was contingent on major or matching funding from state or federal sources. Now, with massive infusions of federal funds stemming from the war on terrorism, virtually every locale in the United States can enhance their emergency capabilities beyond the day-to-day fire and rescue, law enforcement, and EMS responses. Most of the federal funding comes with essential checks and balances to ensure that the funds are spent wisely.

Critical to such funding and other material support is the requirement for comprehensive and viable planning, training, and evaluation of preparedness programs. NIMS, ICS, and other related programs provide today's civic leaders with the essential framework for effective planning and response. However, it takes the specialists and leaders who make up the ES community (the firefighters, law enforcement officers, EMS providers, and emergency planners) to make these plans a reality. Leadership at every level, from the squad up through the state's highest reaches of government, is critical to provide for collective safety.

COLLABORATION BETWEEN MILITARY AND PUBLIC SECTOR EMERGENCY SERVICES ORGANIZATIONS

Proximity to an active military or naval installation is one of the most beneficial circumstances a community can have in the development of a sustained, viable emergency preparedness program. In the United States, from the time when Navy shore installations were first developed, and in later years with the creation of a standing Army and its posts and forts, the military has had a positive influence on most communities well beyond

Table 2-1 List of Cross-Referenced Terms

Former Term		AFIMS Term		NIMS or NRP Term	
WOC	Wing Operations Center	ICC	Installation Control Center	MCS	Multiagency Coordination System
N/A	Battle Staff	CAT	Crisis Action Team	N/A	Crisis Action Team in the Multiagency Coordination Entity
OSC	On Scene Commander (initial)	IC	Incident Commander	IC	Incident Commander
DCG/OSC	Disaster Control Group/On Scene Commander (follow on)	EOC Director	Emergency Operations Center Director		Equivalent to the Mayor, Governor, or Jurisdictional Emergency Management Director in the EOC
DCG	Disaster Control Group	EOC	Emergency Operations Center	EOC	Emergency Operations Center
SRC	Survival Recovery Center	EOC	Emergency Operations Center	EOC	Emergency Operations Center
IRF	Initial Response Force	N/A	First Responders	N/A	First Responders
MCP	Mobile Command Post	Various		Various	
FOE	Follow-On Element	N/A	Emergency Responders	N/A	Emergency Responders
MSCA	Military Support to Civil Authorities	DSCA	Defense Support of Civil Authorities	DSCA	Defense Support of Civil Authorities
RWG	Readiness Working Group	EMWG	Emergency Management Working Group	N/A	N/A
DRF	Disaster Response Force	DRF	Disaster Response Force	N/A	N/A
N/A	Command Post	N/A	Command Post	N/A	Command Post
FSTR Plan 10-2	Full Spectrum Threat Response Plan 10-2	CEMP 10-2	Comprehensive Emergency Management Plan 10-2	EOP	Emergency Operations Plan

Source: U.S. Air Force (2010). Air Force emergency management program. Air Force Instruction 10–2501, p. 20–21.

the immediate economic impact. In times of need, from natural disasters to man-made accidents, the military has always assisted local authorities in coping with the demands of the situation.

Such support, although welcome, is not without its cost, and much to the surprise of some civic leaders, the American military is not charged with supplanting or otherwise replacing the obligations of local governments to develop and manage their own preparedness programs. Even with today's focus on preparedness as part of the war on terrorism, the military role in assisting civil authorities has of necessity become more restricted, caused in part by deployment of vast resources overseas. Foremost in any military unit's obligations to national defense is to maintain its operational capability at virtually any cost. If a commander is faced with the dilemma of assisting civil authorities versus maintaining those operational capabilities, there is no choice but to elect the second option. In today's military services, where funding is increasingly critical, a commander must weigh many options before committing a unit or installation's resources to assisting civil authorities. There likewise exist specific and complex legal issues with which both commanders and local civic leaders must contend. There are legal constraints on how the military can be used in support of civil authorities, particularly for law enforcement, the most notable being the Posse Comitatus Act (10 U.S.C. §375). This prohibits federal military forces from enforcing civilian laws. Such forces may not participate in a search, seizure, arrest, or similar activity in support of local law enforcement, with the exception that state National Guard troops, under the direction of the governor, may do so provided such authority is granted through state laws. But if National Guard forces are called into federal service by the president, they must comply with the restrictions imposed by the Posse Comitatus Act.

However, Congress has enacted a number of statutory provisions by which varying levels of federal military support can be provided to local law enforcement authorities. For example, 10 U.S.C. §371 allows the military to provide local law enforcement officials with any law enforcement information collected "during the normal course of military training or operations." Also, 10 U.S.C. §372 allows the military to loan any equipment, base facility, or research facility to local law enforcement, although it can be made available on a reimbursable basis. In addition, 10 U.S.C. §373 makes military personnel available to train federal, state, and local civilian law enforcement officials on operation and maintenance of military equipment properly loaned per 10 U.S.C. §374, or such military personnel can be assigned to operate such equipment to support local authorities under very limited circumstances.

There is nothing to preclude the military from engaging in humanitarian acts (e.g., in relief of imminent danger situations) consistent with their own operational commitments. However, "... the courts will examine humanitarian acts to ensure the military is not engaging in a subterfuge to disguise a Posse Comitatus Act violation" (U.S. Air Force, 2009, p. 392). This is where real leadership can be demonstrated between the military and public safety. The military, carefully under civilian leadership in Washington, D.C., is starting to take on more of the home mission. Between securing national borders, aiding in recovery from natural disasters, fighting the influx of drugs, and protecting internal infrastructure against terrorism, the military and public safety professionals increasingly work together. The trick is to balance the collaboration so as not to blur the lines too much. The best way to manage this is to have agreements in place that spell out who does what and when. This pre-planning phase can help everyone keep perspective and be the most effective they can be, both individually and collaboratively.

Mutual aid agreements are permissible between federal military units and installations and local civil authorities, subject to a wide range of legal and fiscal constraints. The most common mutual aid agreement is between the fire services of the military and local authorities, in which each can augment the other in times of need. Such situations must adhere to the imminent danger criteria and, even more importantly, must not have an adverse impact on the military's own immediate mission or its resources. Sending fire trucks off base to help contain an industrial fire that threatens to overwhelm the local fire department's abilities and affect the community likely meets the imminent danger criteria, but the commander must ensure that such deployments do not strip the installation of its own essential ES. Installations with flying activities are most acutely aware of this delicate balance, given the potential for accidents and incidents associated with aircraft takeoffs, landings, and local area operations. By extension, EMS capabilities and support may likewise be incorporated into fire department mutual aid agreements or may be the subject of stand-alone agreements with local EMS providers, local hospitals, and other healthcare providers.

Care must also be exercised by commanders in allowing military personnel to assist local authorities on an individual, volunteer basis during and following disasters. First, there is the necessity of maintaining primary mission capabilities, which means having sufficient personnel available to sustain the mission. Second (and this becomes even more important in overseas situations), care must be taken to ensure that such volunteer aid does not jeopardize the legal status of military personnel involved. Most states have enacted Good Samaritan laws to protect volunteers from liabilities arising from their service, provided that they do not exceed the scope of their abilities or any previous training. However, the applicability of Good Samaritan laws may come into question if a military volunteer exceeds (or so someone claims) his or her abilities or previous training. In overseas areas, Status of Forces Agreements usually spell out the status of volunteers or the military's situation relative to humanitarian activities.

The basic guideline, relevant for any ES professional, is that it is the local government's responsibility to provide for the community's well-being in times of disasters and that, subject to mission considerations, the military will assist where feasible and when allowed by law. Some communities, and even states, despite their best plans and programs, can be quickly overwhelmed by events, and in such situations, the military intervenes to get them through the initial crises. Recent examples include the military response to Hurricane Katrina and to the tsunamis in the Southern Pacific region.

The doctrine of imminent danger is a critical point. The military is not normally equipped, organized, or funded to provide long-term support to the civilian community in its recovery efforts. By necessity, unless otherwise directed by higher military authority (usually including funding or on a reimbursable basis) the military can only provide relief of imminent serious conditions. This is typically considered to be the saving of human life, suppression of fires having public safety impact, containment of hazardous materials threatening the community, and preservation of critical public infrastructure (e.g., hospitals, critical communications, public but not private utilities). However, nowhere is the military responsible for the recovery or rehabilitation of civilian property, whether private or government owned, other than National Guard forces acting under the direction of the state's governor and funded for such activity. Once the immediate crisis is under control, the military (again, with the possible exception of the National Guard) returns to base to resume its normal activities.

CONCLUSION

Current and emerging ES plans, procedures, protocols, command and control, organizations, and planning and implementation processes are rooted in military history. Many ES leaders have had military experience at various levels, which was readily applied to the civilian sector. Even if they have not served in the military, current and emerging leaders have been able to adapt a military model in enhancing their organizational responses to the outside world. Using their military experience or being able to adopt the more positive aspects of the military by nonveterans has enabled ES leaders to forge much more effective organizations.

The fire service leaders in the United States played a major role in the development and dissemination of more comprehensive, viable approaches to command and control, planning, and organization of the ES community both at home and abroad. Such programs are again rooted in military planning for the ultimate disaster—that of warfare—and the innumerable events that might comprise readiness to defend the nation. With the global war on terror in full swing, there has been a necessarily closer spirit of cooperation between the civilian and military hierarchy to ensure national security and preparedness, extending all the way down to the smallest political subdivision and organization.

Wrap-Up

ACTIVITY

Answer the following questions.

1. Implementation of ICS would be appropriate for what kind of incident?

2. What steps can preparedness organizations take to help implement NIMS?

3. Why are NIMS exercises an important part of successful NIMS implementation?

4. Describe the main role of MACS.

5. Discuss the relationship between NIMS and the National Response Plan.

6. What are some of the federal or state military resources in your jurisdiction's area that might be called on to assist you if your resources are overwhelmed?

7. What are some of your resources that a nearby state or federal military installation or activity might call on if needed?

8. When was the last time you held an exercise that included the state or federal military resources in your area of responsibility?

REFERENCES

Brunacini, A.V. (1985). *Fire command.* Quincy, MA: National Fire Protection Association.

Chase, R. A. (1980). *FIRESCOPE: A new concept in multiagency fire suppression coordination.* Berkeley, CA: Pacific Southwest Forest and Range Experiment Station. Retrieved from http://www.fs.fed.us/psw/publications/documents/psw_gtr040/psw_gtr040.pdf

Covey, S. R. (2004). *The 8th habit: From effectiveness to greatness.* New York, NY: Free Press.

Federal Emergency Management Agency. (2004a). *NIMS and the Incident Command System.* Retrieved from http://www.fema.gov/txt/nims/nims_ics_position_paper.txt

Federal Emergency Management Agency. (2004b). IS-700 *National Incident Management System, an introduction.* Retrieved from http://training.fema.gov/EMIWEB/IS/is700.asp

Irwin, B. (1981). FIRESCOPE: A record of the significant decisions. Retrieved from http://www.firescope.org/firescope-history/Some%20Highlights%20of%20the%20Evolution%20of%20the%20ICS.pdf

U.S. Air Force. (2007). *Emergency management*. Air Force Policy Directive 10-25. USAF Judge Advocate General's school. *The Military Commander and the Law.* Maxwell AFB AL: AFJAGS Press.

U.S. Air Force. (2009). *The military commander and the law*. Retrieved from http://www.airforcewriter.com/Military_CC_and_Law2009_Pdf

U.S. Air Force. (2010). *Air Force emergency management program*. Air Force Instruction 10-2501. USAF Judge Advocate General's school. *The Military Commander and the Law.* Maxwell AFB AL: AFJAGS Press.

Walsh, D., Christen, H., Miller, G., Callsen, C., Cilluffo, F., & Maniscalco, P. (2005). *National incident management system: Principles and practice*. Sudbury, MA: Jones and Bartlett Publishers.

Other Considerations for Emergency Services Leaders

Chris Nollette and Frank P. Nollette

On September 11, 2001, New York City Mayor Rudy Giuliani became a visible and active leader as he and his personnel managed the aftermath of the terrorist attacks. However, what many may not know is that long before these unfathomable events occurred, Mayor Giuliani had applied several key management strategies. Those strategies enhanced his ability to lead the city that day and in the days that followed. Mayor Giuliani held morning meetings with the chiefs of his key departments. After becoming mayor, he evaluated who attended these meetings and who really needed to attend. Department heads who were held down by several layers of bureaucracy on the city's organizational chart where elevated, or new departments were created to bring these people to the table. In a 2002 article entitled Leadership, *Mayor Giuliani emphasized asking "what the mission is" (p. 306) and who needs a "seat at the table," (p. 309), in order to make planning easier and to respond with a proactive mindset—not just a reactive one. His leadership approach even had a humanistic side, demonstrated by the many funerals he attended of the responders who perished on September 11. He tells the story of how his father instilled this "weddings discretionary, funerals mandatory" (pp. 253–264) mentality and how it is more important to honor and respect the fallen and their survivors than it is to celebrate a new beginning.*

INTRODUCTION

Perhaps the patch worn on a uniform or the badge on a chest becomes the shield that distinguishes current leaders as modern-day warriors. Why do some in the emergency services willingly accept the full weight of responsibility, whereas others shrink from a leadership role? This chapter examines leadership tools that every leader should consider as part of an overall leadership toolkit. Successful leaders know that planning and preparation are key to effective operations. Although planning may seem like more of a management topic, it is also a critical component of successful leadership. Like the approach that Mayor Giuliani used, without proper planning processes, the leader's vision remains simply a

vision. This chapter also addresses the emotional and physiological aspects of leadership and offers suggestions for recognizing and coping with stress and maintaining a healthy lifestyle. Leaders may be technically competent but still fail to lead effectively because they are overwhelmed by stress or lack of sleep.

THE IMPORTANCE OF PLANNING

There are countless means and methods for executing the planning function. Finding the planning methods that work best takes time, study, and experimentation. It is unlikely that a single method covers all aspects of planning in an organization. For example, more complex planning is needed when working on a project to cut response times to alarms or 911 calls, or to implement a revised prehospital protocol. Revising a county's mass casualty plans to accommodate new federal mandates and a loss of state funding demands even more complex analysis and planning. The more complex the goals, the more complex the planning, and herein is one of the first essential steps in planning: goal setting.

Goal setting can take place through a variety of means, from conferences to brain storming sessions to the hiring of outside consultants and contractors. Some goals likely are established and communicated downward from a higher authority, and the designated leader is required to do whatever it takes to meet these goals. Some goals fall within the leader's purview to establish independently. In either scenario, an effective leader never stops planning, because there are always different, new, or better ways of doing things. More importantly, any planning must of necessity be dynamic. Circumstances or premises of a plan may change dramatically, in some cases overnight or in an even shorter time frame.

Early in 2010, Haiti was struck by catastrophic earthquakes. Many nations rushed aid to the affected region. Relief groups encountered problems initially because of the lack of adequate air terminal facilities and air traffic control, plus a lack of reliable communications within the country. These problems were eventually sorted out, and aid began to flow much more rapidly. The fact that the aid began to flow in a relatively short time is a testament to the foresight and planning of many individuals, organizations, and governments. Shortly thereafter, Chile was struck by massive earthquakes, and whatever plans that nation and the nations willing to provide aid had in place were severely tested, because the magnitude of the disaster exceeded all expectations. For the nations providing aid, new plans had to be developed and implemented on the fly, because most organizations did not envision having to cope with two major disasters geographically distant from one another and from the assisting nations. Complicating this response scenario was the fact that Haiti and Chile each had different needs initially and in the long term, and the nations offering assistance had finite resources. Because of effective planning by the leadership of all of the organizations and governments involved, utter chaos was avoided and recovery efforts were able to move forward.

In any organization, but especially in the emergency services arena, planning is essential to sustain ongoing levels of service and productivity and achieve the organization's goals. Perhaps one of the most daunting tasks is to determine what needs to be done, if indeed something needs to be done. Changes in laws, rules, regulations, or protocols all require planning to accommodate the changes. This involves more than just the leader, because no effective planning can take place without the active participation of others. One problem area for leaders is the temptation to work through planning phases independently. In very small organizations, there may be little choice and the leader must do all or most of the planning. Usually, however, there are others within and outside the organization who can and should be allowed to participate in planning. This is where the concept of synergy is manifested: the combined knowledge and intelligence of the participants yields a product of far greater value than the simple sum of the parts. Trying to plan alone raises the very real risk of overlooking critical points, or even unconsciously allowing one's own biases to interfere with this essential step in an organization's development, growth, and sustainability.

Restricting the number of people involved in the planning process may be necessary in some instances, because of security and confidentiality constraints. For example, knowledge of the details of how an agency plans to respond to a terrorist biological attack is, of necessity, restricted to those with a need to know. This illustrates a dilemma of planning, especially of contingency planning: How much detail does one include in the plan? Ideally, such plans should provide broad direction to the various agencies or work units, rather than comprehensive how-to-do-it details. Police, fire, and emergency medical services (EMS) responders are relied on to know what has to be done when they are on scene, so the details of their regular tasks need not be in the plan.

Inherent in planning is identifying measurable steps in the implementation process and the means to assess progress or success. A professor of decision-making analysis was once overheard to make the very trenchant statement that, "...to some people, movement in any direction is considered progress." It is hoped that movement in this instance is in a positive direction, but that assumes there is some method in place to assess both the direction and magnitude of such movement. How does one know if goals have been achieved?

Imagine a department has been asked to cut response times to 911 calls. How does one know whether the measures implemented to achieve this goal have been effective? Statistical analysis of response times over a given period of time, compared to historical records, is the prime indicator of success, but the situation can be looked at in more detail. What is driving the goal? How do the response times compare to those of other jurisdictions? Are there any mandated federal, state, or local standards for response times, and if so, how does the department measure up against them? This presupposes that (1) adequate historical data are available for comparison; (2) there is a means of capturing current data in a timely manner and in a format that allows comparison; and (3) any changes in policies, procedures, or protocols to improve response times are positive in nature.

The third point bears a bit more discussion. Response times can be quickly improved by driving faster. However, factor in the many other issues that driving faster raises. The leader must consider the potential for accidents en route to the scene and the increased potential for liability this brings, the added wear and tear on the vehicle fleet, the increased fuel consumption from driving at higher speeds, whether drivers are adequately trained to drive at higher speeds, and so forth. Is improving response time actually a positive change that will benefit the organization and the population it serves? Can this approach be sustained in a cost-effective manner? If voters fail to approve a municipal bond package that would have financed the building, equipping, and staffing of two new fire stations to serve a growing population affected by urban sprawl, how would that affect the goal?

Many leaders are astounded at just how complex planning really is when they actually participate in the process. One can attend college courses or specialized training, sometimes service-specific, in public administration and management to learn the theories, tools, and techniques of planning. Independent research and study likewise can add to the leader's arsenal of resources. Any and all of these give leaders the essential tools to use in a planning effort, but not until one actually starts active planning does the magnitude of the process become apparent.

Leadership Points to Ponder

Vision without proper planning is only a dream.

Planning by the Five Rs

There are five aspects of the planning process: (1) requirements, (2) resources, (3) responses, (4) research, and (5) reality. Each of these elements has direct and immediate application to planning, particularly in the emergency response realm. For any planning effort, all five come into play, and there is no sharp dividing line between them, because they inevitably overlap.

Requirements

A good plan starts with two essential questions:

■ Why is the plan needed?

■ What are the plan's requirements?

Without adequately answering these questions, one does not know how to proceed. Hastily developed requirements typically lead to, at best, confusing or conflicting plans and programs. This does not imply that everything needs a detailed plan, because sudden changes in a given situation may require immediate action without the benefit of a planning period. The battalion chief on the fireground, the lieutenant leading a SWAT team, or the senior paramedic coordinating triage in a mass casualty event does not have the luxury of stopping everything to develop a more comprehensive plan. Furthermore, plans developed to meet stated requirements should not be so rigid that there is no latitude for action in changing circumstances. The plan should provide essential guidance for responders without preventing them from achieving the intended outcomes.

Requirements can be thought of as risks. What are the threats or risks within the community or assigned area of operations and responsibility? The community or agency should have records of past experiences with risks that typically recur in the local area or have a chance of occurring on a less frequent basis. Such records can be invaluable to the planner. In many parts of the nation, for example, it is virtually certain that winter will bring heavy snow, white-out conditions, and freezing temperatures, so the emergency service agencies in those areas are well prepared to cope with this seasonal risk. A sudden winter storm with ice and sleet occurring in a warmer region may find that area ill-prepared for such weather because it occurs so rarely.

Resources

After the requirements are sufficiently identified, the planner must determine what resources, such as equipment, facilities, staffing, and funding, are required to execute the plan under development as well as what resources are available. Note that requirements may have to be altered to match resources, or vice versa, because planning is, of necessity, a dynamic process. The resources of neighboring organizations, agencies, and government sources at all levels should be considered; knowing what the neighbors have can help one make much more realistic plans if there are provisions in place to call for these assets. Preexisting mutual aid agreements can be of tremendous value if properly researched, written, agreed to, and exercised to ensure that they are indeed workable. However, dependence on outside resources is a risky strategy and can leave a community vulnerable to potentially disastrous outcomes. Ideally, each community should have sufficient resources to cope with disaster situations and the day-to-day provision of essential public safety services. In the aftermath of the terrorist attacks of 9/11, the sudden availability of federal funds to state, county, and city governments allowed many to completely revitalize their programs with new equipment, training, recruiting, and a myriad of things long sought but previously unaffordable.

Planners cannot allow themselves to think of resources only in terms of equipment, structures, or funds. The human element is also a critical consideration. The use of volunteers and nongovernmental organizations can fill many staffing gaps, particularly in protracted responses that last days or even weeks and months. Cultivating positive relationships with nongovernmental organizations and volunteer organizations can go a long way toward giving an agency the qualified, well-trained people it needs to carry out its missions.

When budgeting for resources, it is helpful to map out several options at increasing levels of investment. The following levels provide a rough guideline:

- Mandated or minimum essential services at the most basic level
- The above minimums plus some additional or enhanced services that are economically feasible with a positive cost–benefit ratio
- All of the above plus supplemental resources that the organization would like to have, again meeting the standard of a positive cost–benefit ratio

Determining just what the absolute minimum services are and their true cost is complicated, especially for larger jurisdictions, and may require assistance from local or state financial departments, other agencies, or independent contractors.

Leadership Points to Ponder

Like the 300 Spartans at The Battle of Thermopylae who were outnumbered by the Persian Army 1000 to 1, responders are usually outnumbered by the number of patients at major incidents. Having a dynamic plan for additional resources is imperative for leaders.

Responses

The measure of an agency's planning is the quality of its responses. A flawed response to a major event all too quickly makes evident any shortcomings in agency resources, inadequacies in responder capabilities, and, more importantly, errors in planning. Postresponse critiques at all levels are invaluable in understanding these variables. The most effective postincident critiques are held in brainstorming fashion, wherein no blame is made and no fingers are pointed, but an open and honest discussion is held to identify how the system or plans failed to meet the expectations of all involved. From such discussions, plans can be revised, resources reallocated, additional training and education provided, and other needs addressed.

Caution must be exercised in the degree to which an agency reveals such critiques to the public or other outsiders, because the information can too easily be turned into a potent weapon that can adversely affect the agency's credibility. To someone on the outside looking in who does not know the full scope of the event and any issues that arose, and does not understand just how or why something did or did not occur, it is too easy to affix blame without a coherent rationale.

Research

Research may be the starting point in developing plan requirements, and it may be used to figure out how to meet plan requirements. Research can encompass a wide variety of sources and, in some instances, may require outside expertise. As a short case study, look at the challenge of providing services to a growing population in an urban environment. Where does one start?

It is usually easier to start with the known and work to the unknown. So what is known about the situation? A lot of information likely can be drawn from one's own agency's existing plans and programs, plus any historical data that can be found. Someone must be tasked with rooting through files, archives, or even city, county, or state records to gain a feel for what once was and what is now occurring. Another good research strategy is to find out what other area agencies are doing or what best practices exist nationwide for districts of this size and demographic profile. What services do they provide? How do they deliver those services? Have they developed any innovative programs that emphasize prevention? If so, could the agency adopt a similar program to improve outcomes for the community?

Statistical analysis can be revealing if one has the data, the instruments or programs to massage that data, and the expertise to interpret the findings. In government agencies, there are likely a lot of folks in the planning department and various other divisions who have that expertise. Nearby college or universities have seniors and graduate students in statistics, public administration and policy, healthcare management, and related programs who would revel in the chance to work on a real-world research project. A polite inquiry to the appropriate faculty department head will net more help than can be imagined, all at minimal cost to the agency. It might be necessary to write an evaluation of each student's work at the end of the project, or to provide desk space and computer access. In some instances, paid internships may be possible, again working through the appropriate faculty adviser.

Finally, the power of documentation cannot be overstated. Whatever is learned should be written down. Information gathered should be put into one coherent research document that members of the team, administration officials, and other stakeholders can review and discuss. Not only does this show that the team has done its homework, but it is also a valuable resource for the future as new recruits face the next generation of planning challenges.

Reality

The planning process can create tunnel vision, because the plans seem to take on a life of their own. It is critical that planners step back from the work periodically and ensure that what is being proposed and developed is indeed within the realm of possibility. Fire, law enforcement, and medical agencies in Tucson, Arizona, do not have to factor the possibility of a tsunami into their emergency plans as do their counterparts in Hilo, Hawaii. Or do they? It's unlikely that a tsunami will ever hit Tucson. But what if one hits the coast of Southern

California and local, state, or federal agencies activate mutual aid agreements? These agreements might require that Tucson dispatch specialized teams of firefighters, police, or emergency medical technicians and paramedics to California, which in turn would affect resource availability in Tucson while these people and equipment are deployed. So Tucson does not plan for tsunamis, but they do plan for deploying their people and resources in a mutual aid agreement. They also plan for providing continuing service to the population with a realignment of the remaining resources when deployments are made.

In an industrial area, the fire, police, and medical services plan for (and it is hoped exercise) their response procedures and protocols according to the hazards or threats posed by the environment. If an explosion releases toxic gases or hazardous particulate materials into the atmosphere, the chances of containing all of that material are virtually nonexistent. Responding agencies need to direct the evacuation of people in the danger zone; provide rescue, aid, and comfort to the injured; minimize further damage (perhaps fires); and otherwise isolate the area until remedial actions can be implemented. Thus, the response plans must reflect the reality of what a worst-case scenario would look like versus the ideal of being able to completely contain the incident.

PHYSIOLOGICAL AND EMOTIONAL FACTORS IN EMERGENCY SERVICES LEADERSHIP

One of the areas that leaders and managers have historically failed to address is human resources. Our personnel are the keys that make or break leaders. Our personnel are constantly working under less than ideal conditions and experience many hardships that include stress, sleep deprivation, and emotional issues. These same stressors were experienced by you, the leader, as you ascended the professional career ladder (or will be if you are starting to climb that ladder). As we become leaders in our organizations, we must deal with a number of issues that challenge our abilities to lead. The stress of the job exponentially grows as we take on more responsibilities.

Stress carries many physiological and emotional ramifications if not controlled. We not only have to learn to deal with stress, but we are also obligated as leaders to assist our personnel in understanding its affects on us and managing it properly. Stress can lead to sleep deprivation, which carries another set of problems. However, before we can effectively deal with these stressors, we must seek our own internal gauges. Knowing oneself, and addressing our own weaknesses, is paramount to being a successful leader. Without taking that inward look, we cannot properly lead our followers to do the same.

Stress

Stress is a powerful force that influences performance at every level, including cognitive (thinking), psychomotor (hands-on), and affective (emotion). To a large extent, the level of stress that leaders experience during the direst circumstances determines how successful they will be personally and professionally. The most effective way to minimize the body's natural stress response is through mental and physical conditioning over time, particularly repeated drills and exposure to situations and scenarios. Extensive studies have been conducted on how best to train military forces and police officers to control their use of deadly force in very stressful situations. The results indicate that when people practice and rehearse their reactions over and over, making responses instinctive rather than dependent on conscious thought, they are able to function at a higher level under stress. To understand why this is effective, one must explore the physiology of the human stress response.

Stress has little effect on gross motor skills, such as walking, running, or jumping. This allows humans to flee when threatened by immediate harm. Where stress does come into play is on the fine motor side. Stress puts a person into a hyperactive state, which overwhelms fine motor skills and impairs hand–eye coordination, both of which are essential in patient care, among other things. In addition to the loss of fine motor skills, there is a measurable loss of cognitive ability (Siddle, 2008).

The effects of stress on performance have led researchers to coin the phrase the "inverted-U hypothesis." In his book *Sharpening the Warrior's Edge: The Psychology & Science of Training*, Siddle (2008) notes:

> . . . The Inverted-U Hypothesis simply proposes that increases in arousal are accompanied in the quality of performance up to a certain point, after which additional increases in arousal result in deterioration in the quality of performance.

This phenomenon was first demonstrated in mice with experiments designed and conducted by Robert Yerkes and John Dodson, the results of which were published in 1908 in the *Journal of Comparative Neurology and Psychology*. Researchers Weinberg, Gould, and Jackson (1979) later applied this pioneering work to humans and found in separate studies that, at particular levels of stress, a certain amount of cognitive and motor ability is lost. When the human body perceives stress, the production of adrenaline (also known as epinephrine) increases dramatically and causes an increase in blood supply. This allows large muscles to work more effectively, but it produces the opposite effect in smaller, finer muscles. In addition, heart rate increases and breathing quickens, muscles tighten, and hearing becomes more acute while the field of vision narrows.

Researchers have noted that heartbeat can be used to determine stress level. When the heartbeat climbs above 145 beats per minute there is a definite loss of fine motor skills and complex performance, whereas gross motor functions increase. This can be attributed to the sympathetic nervous system response called "fight or flight," a term coined by Harvard doctor and physiologist Walter Bradford Cannon in 1915. During the fight or flight response, large muscle groups must harness an incredible amount of strength to overcome a life-or-death event.

Siddle (2008) addresses the physiology of this response as follows:

> . . . First, as the heart rate increases, the visual system adjusts to deal with the threat by limiting the amount of information the brain receives. Second, the brain's normal ability to process (analyze and evaluate) a wide range of information quickly is focused to specific items. Therefore, additional clues which would normally be processed are either lost or misinterpreted. If the stress is perceived as spontaneous and overwhelming, hypervigilance occurs.

The body is in survival mode and must decide quickly whether to run or to stay and fight. Resources the body considers unnecessary in this state, notably fine motor skills and cognitive ability, are sacrificed to channel all available energy into one's capacity to escape the crisis or attack the threat. Although this primitive response serves well in certain circumstances, it can be a severe handicap during situations that require complex thinking and dexterity, such as the need to intubate a critically injured child at a disaster scene with a hysterical mother nearby. Stress that continues to escalate out of control can lead to hypervigilance, a state in which individuals are stuck in a loop, constantly redoing a task over and over, or paralysis, simply shutting down and unable to move.

Over time, sustained adrenaline highs damage one's physical and mental status to the point where they are unable to perform at any level. There have been numerous accounts of soldiers, especially in the first and second World wars who fought for weeks or months without respite and then suffered a physical or mental collapse. It may take hours to come down from the effects of the adrenaline that is pumped into the bloodstream during stressful incidents. Individuals may have "the shakes" and may have trouble sleeping.

Strategies for Controlling Stress

Leaders must make an effort to prevent being controlled by stress. Controlling stress is not difficult, but so many fail to use even the simplest of strategies and allow the stress to build up. When this happens, leaders can be thrown off their game and do and say things that they normally would not. Researchers have noted that most doctors' visits can be traced back to the amount of stress that individuals are experiencing. It is known that stress can lead to emotional problems, a lack of concentration, memory loss, irritability, mood swings, and depression. It has long been noted that increased stress can cause a variety of illnesses, ranging from simple headaches to heart attacks. To become an effective leader, one should consider the following steps to help reduce stress to a healthier level.

Leadership Points to Ponder

[Sleep is] the golden chain that ties health and our bodies together.

Thomas Dekker

(from *http://www.quotationspage.com*)

Sleep

Adequate sleep is essential for effective functioning, especially for anyone serving in the emergency services. Yet, it has become a badge of honor in modern society, especially among public safety professionals and the military, to deny the critical need for sleep. People are indeed sleeping less. In 1960, the American Cancer Society surveyed 1 million Americans and found that people slept an average of 8 hours per night. Dr. Diane Elliot and Dr. Kerry Kuehl, (2007), associate professors of medicine at Oregon Health Sciences University, cited that Americans have dropped to just 6.7 hours of sleep per night. Many in public safety and the military would argue that theirs is even lower than this on a daily basis. Eve Van Cauter, an endocrinologist at the University of Chicago School of Medicine, notes, "Four to six hours of sleep [per night] in just six days puts one on the road to a pre-diabetic state . . . contributing to an epidemic of obesity" (Spiegel, Leproult, & Van Cauter, 1999). The release of the hormone leptin caused by sleep deprivation is to blame, and as people put on more weight, they are at increased risk of more than 30 different medical conditions that can be lethal. The science of sleep is generally not well understood or respected by leaders in public safety. An examination of the different sleep stages provides a clearer picture of the role sleep plays in health.

Sleep is broadly segmented into rapid eye movement (REM) and non-REM sleep. Non-REM sleep is further divided into four stages. The first two stages lead to deep sleep, which then occurs during stages three and four. These last two stages are particularly critical for health. One essentially sinks into a mini-coma, enabling the body to devote its energy to repairing tissue damage at the cellular level, including heart and lung tissue. If people awaken during this mini-coma, they commonly experience sleep inertia, meaning difficulty falling back to sleep, and bodily repairs do not continue until the following night. Over time, the cumulative effects of such disturbances in sleep or lack of sleep can be devastating. There is increased risk of heart and lung disease, cancer, depression, and hypertension. This risk, although centered on personal health, becomes even more compelling when the men and women of public safety and the military have an additional responsibility: the protection of others.

The REM stage of sleep is known as the dream state. This sleep pattern allows the body to process thoughts and emotions experienced during the day and to restore mental health. Generally, when bodies are functioning well, they naturally regulate the time spent in REM and non-REM sleep, depending on the degree to which the specialized repairs each stage provides are needed.

People who are chronically sleep deprived (e.g., people who chronically consume too much alcohol) often do not sense their limitations. They believe that they have trained themselves to function with limited sleep. Sleep research indicates otherwise. In one study, Matthew Walker (2007), director of the Sleep and Neuroimaging Laboratory at the University of California, Berkeley, took a group of young college undergraduates and deprived them of sleep for 35 hours straight. Walker then placed them in a magnetic resonance imaging scanner and showed them increasingly negative and disturbing images. Although the control group showed moderate and controlled responses in the emotional centers of their brains, the sleep-deprived group showed a hyperactive brain response. Walker (2007) noted that when these brain scans were compared to scans from patients who had psychiatric disorders, the images were impossible to differentiate.

Elliott and Kuehl (2007) note that a person who misses just one night of sleep suffers from reduced psychomotor vigilance (meaning the ability to respond quickly to a visual stimulus), and their thinking is impaired by as much as 40%. When sleep deprivation becomes chronic, even after just several nights, increased accidents and depression can be added to the mix. If this is not scary enough consider that, according to Elliott and Kuehl (2007), averaging fewer than 6 hours of sleep a night for 6 days is similar in effect to smoking a pack of cigarettes a day.

Statistics on the effects of sleep deprivation and disruption in various professions are equally sobering. In November 2006, the *Journal of Occupational and Environmental Medicine* published a meta-analysis of 32 studies that showed an increase in testicular cancer, prostate cancer, and lymphomas in those who were chronically sleep deprived (Sheedy, 2006). In March 2007, the *New England Journal of Medicine* reported that the leading cause of death for firefighters is not on-scene incidents during the line of duty, but rather heart disease (Kales, Soteriades, Christophi, & Christiani, 2007). In December 2007, the prestigious medical journal *The Lancet* reported that a World Health Organization study on nurses and firefighters who worked night shifts showed that they experienced increased rates of colon, prostate, and breast cancer (Straif, et al., 2007). This should be a wake-up call for anyone who fails to monitor their sleep patterns and get between 6.5 and 8 hours of sleep a night. The evidence continues to mount that sleep is critical for on-the-job performance and long-term health, and leaders must make sure they address this need for themselves and their staff on a daily basis.

Exercise

Exercise is often overlooked by people in leadership positions. Bodies were made to be used, and over time humans have become more sedentary, which further inhibits mental and physical health. Leaders who are usually under stress must participate in at least some level of physical activity each and every day. There has been a tremendous amount of research showing that failure to exercise puts one in great danger of cardiovascular and respiratory diseases. Exercise does not have to be tremendously rigorous to be beneficial but should be enough to get the heart rate up to the target zone. Leaders should make it a part of their daily routine to do some manner of exercise, even if it is a simple walk through the park. The time that one spends exercising can also be a time for self-reflection, to get a clearer picture of the problems that are faced on a daily basis. This time allows the body to work off some of the adrenaline that is pumped into the veins by the body as a natural response to stress. Burning off some of this excess can bring down the heart rate, relax the body, and allow leaders to think more clearly and thus solve problems and face challenges. This simple step, in combination with proper sleep, allows the leader to manage stress to an acceptable level.

Diet

The food one eats is critical to success. For many people, diets contain more calories than needed and may not be balanced nutritionally. Some modest changes, such as a decrease in sugary drinks and more attention to sodium intake, and a slight adjustment to caloric intake, will make a difference in overall health and allow one to manage stress. Recent news reports have emphasized that America may be on the brink of a prediabetes epidemic. This epidemic of obesity is causing great concern among health professionals and is showing up at younger and younger ages, which should be a warning to all Americans. Small changes to one's diet may have a significant impact on overall health, and this may significantly reduce stress.

Leadership Points to Ponder

Emotions are contagious. Our social skills depend on responding and anticipating the actions or intents of others. We become social chameleons.

Socialization

It has long been known that humans are social beings; the support and wisdom of others is needed to help navigate the trials and tribulations of life. Yet so many leaders live their lives in a vacuum and bring very few (if any) others into their inner circles. When leaders isolate themselves, it can lead to changes in their mental and physical state of being. These changes can have adverse and long-term results that reduce their effectiveness. Too many leaders believe that they can "go it alone," only to find that the going can be much harder than what they bargained for, leaving them depressed and isolated. These stressful feelings continue to erode the effectiveness of the leader and bring about more stress. Socialization is the key to sharing with others the burden of simply living. Talking with others allows one to gain perspective on problems and can lead to more clarity on how to proceed.

Although stress is a normal part of life, too much can be damaging and can have negative physical and emotional consequences. Leaders must take steps to manage their stress, and simple steps can have a huge payoff for leaders and those who depend on them. The problem must be addressed, so that leaders can continue to build their emotional and social intelligence, which is the cornerstone of their effectiveness.

CONCLUSION

Effective leadership depends on practical considerations as much as it does on vision and passion. Without proper planning, visions cannot be implemented. Planning is a complex process that requires a great deal of research and input from others. Leaders who attempt to travel this path alone usually fail at leadership, as it takes at least two people to lead: a leader and a follower.

In addition to looking outward to the health and proper functioning of their organizations, leaders must look inward to their own health and emotional well-being. The emergency services professions are high-stress professions because we are perpetually responding to others' crises. Regular exercise, proper nutrition, adequate sleep, and stress management are the foundations on which leaders can build their success and set a positive example for their staffs. As in the story about Mayor Giuliani highlighted at the beginning of this chapter, leaders who properly plan and treat themselves with dignity and respect can overcome forces much greater than themselves.

3

Wrap-Up

ACTIVITY

Leaders need to score themselves using the international Epworth Sleepiness Scale to determine their risk level, so they can make changes to ensure a healthier lifestyle (TABLE 3-1).

If any of the following are true for you, you are at high risk for a sleep disorder:

- You score greater than 16 on the Epworth Sleepiness Scale.

- You snore.

- You suffer from fatigue-related crashes.

- You are overweight or obese.

- Your neck is greater than 17 inches in circumference.

- You have high blood pressure.

Table 3-1 Epworth Sleepiness Scale

	Never dose off——————————————➤Doze off			
Sit and read	0	1	2	3
Watch TV	0	1	2	3
Sit and talk	0	1	2	3
Ride in car	0	1	2	3
Lying down	0	1	2	3
After lunch	0	1	2	3
Sitting in traffic	0	1	2	3
During a lecture of meeting	0	1	2	3

REFERENCES

Elliot, D. L., & Kuehl, K. S. (2007, June). *The effects of sleep deprivation on fire fighters and EMS responders: Final report.* Fairfax, VA: International Association of Fire Chiefs (IAFC) and the United States Fire Administration (USFA), with assistance from the faculty of Oregon Health & Science University. Retrieved from http://www.iafc.org/files/progsSleep_SleepDeprivationReport.pdf

Giuliani, R. W. (2002). *Leadership.* New York, NY: Hyperion.

Kales, S. N., Soteriades, E. S., Christophi, C., & Christiani, D. C. (2007, March 22). Emergency duties and deaths from heart disease among firefighters in the United States. *New England Journal of Medicine, 356*(12), 1207–1215. Retrieved from http://www.nejm.org/doi/full/10.1056/NEJMoa060357

Sheedy, G. (2006). Training pathways for occupational medicine. *Journal of Occupational and Environmental Medicine, 48*(11), 1113–1115.

Siddle, B. K. (2008). *Sharpening the warrior's edge: The psychology & science of training.* Millstadt, IL: Warrior Science Group.

Spiegel, K., Leproult, R., & Van Cauter, E. (1999). Impact of sleep debt on metabolic and endocrine function. *The Lancet, 354,* 1435–1439.

Straif, K., Baan, R., Grosse, Y., Secretan, B., El Ghissassi, F., Bouvard, V., . . . Cogliano, V. (2007, December). Carcinogenicity of shift-work, painting, and fire-fighting. *The Lancet Oncology, 8*(12), 1065–1066.

Walker, M. (2007). The human emotional brain without sleep—A prefrontal amygdala disconnect. *Current Biology, 17*(20), R877–R878.

Weinberg, R., Gould, D., & Jackson, A. (1979). Expectations and performance: An empirical test of Bandura's self-efficacy theory. *Journal of Sport Psychology, 1*(4), 320–331.

Yerkes, R. M., & Dodson, J. D. (1908, November). The relation of strength of stimulus to rapidity of habit-formation. *Journal of Comparative Neurology and Psychology, 18*(5), 459–482.

Leadership Theory

4

Leader-Centric Theories

Brent J. Goertzen

Leadership is about capacity: the capacity of leaders to listen and observe, to use their expertise as a starting point to encourage dialogue at all levels of decision-making, to establish processes and transparency in decision-making, to articulate their own values and visions clearly but not impose them. Leadership is about setting and not just reacting to agendas, identifying problems, and initiating change that makes for substantial improvement rather than managing change.

Dr. Ann Marie E. McSwain (from *http://www.Medpedia.com*; Professional Summary)

INTRODUCTION

This chapter examines early leadership theories that focus nearly exclusively on the leader. More specifically, trait theory defines a leader by describing the attributes or qualities of individuals who ascended to positions of authority. The leader behavior theory centers on the leader's actions.

The trait approach was one of the first methods that systematically examined leadership. Stogdill's (1948) pioneering work described typical qualities of leaders. He sought to identify a universal set of traits that are common to leaders across all situations. However, he found that there was no consistent set of traits that differentiated leaders from nonleaders across contexts. Still, the trait approach has generated a substantial amount of interest. Even today, researchers seek to explain how traits influence leadership processes.

Research conducted at the Ohio State University and University of Michigan during the 1950s and 1960s ushered in the examination of activities that "leaders do" to enhance employee satisfaction and performance. Early research in leader behaviors has heavily influenced more recent studies in leadership. Even now, scholars are examining various behavioral patterns of leaders and how they help facilitate organizational outcomes. Beyond describing early leadership research, this chapter also describes more contemporary approaches of scholars to describe the unique attributes (e.g., emotional intelligence) and behaviors (e.g., influence tactics) of leaders.

TRAIT THEORIES

Over the years, trait theory as it relates to the understanding of leadership has been a hotly debated topic. For much of the nineteenth century and the first half of the twentieth century, it was a common belief that leaders are born and not made. For instance, Thomas Carlyle's book *Heroes and Hero Worship* (1907), based in part on earlier work by Galton (1869), focused on the importance of heredity as part of what endowed "great men" with "innate" characteristics that shape human personality and behavior. This section examines several of these early trait models and offers contemporary perspectives of characteristics that can affect a leaders' ability to engage with followers.

The earliest social and behavioral research regarding leadership examined the qualities of leaders. Although the term "leadership" was not commonly defined, many of the early studies presumed it to be a process to achieve organizational goals because it "implies activity, movement, getting work done" (Stogdill, 1948, p. 64). It was not uncommon for the research to examine leader characteristics of those holding positions of authority in organizations, but some studies did examine the attributes of individuals who emerged as leaders within newly formed work groups. As such, the early research examined the characteristics of leaders compared to nonleaders.

Stogdill (1948) reviewed all research examining the qualities of individuals who ascended to leadership positions. This review included more than 120 research studies published between 1904 and 1948. He reported five general categories of traits:

- Capacity: Personal traits such as intelligence, communication skills, alertness, and judgment.
- Achievement: Qualities of scholarship and knowledge.
- Responsibility: Traits of dependability, initiative, persistence, self-confidence, and desire to excel.
- Participation: Characteristics of activity, sociability, cooperation, adaptability, and humor.
- Status: Qualities of socioeconomic position and popularity.

Stogdill (1948) also asserted that persons do not become leaders simply by displaying a pattern of characteristics. He noted that leaders in some situations are not necessarily effective in other situations; the situation affects one's ability to lead others in the achievement of organizational goals. His research identified possible situational characteristics that affect leadership, including the followers' knowledge, social status, skills, interests and needs of followers, and objectives to be achieved.

Although this early research was intended to identify a pattern of leader characteristics, Stogdill explained that leadership "appears . . . to be a working relationship among members of a group, in which the leader acquires

status through active participation and demonstration of his or her capacity for carrying cooperative tasks through completion" (Stogdill, 1948, p. 66).

Stogdill (1974) conducted another review of leadership research that included 163 new studies published between 1949 and 1970. This review included many more managerial studies and many more traits that were likely to be associated with leader effectiveness:

- Intelligence and ability: Includes intelligence, judgment and decisiveness, knowledge, and fluency of speech.
- Personality: Includes adjustments (adaptability), aggressiveness and assertiveness, alertness, ascendance, emotional balance, enthusiasm, extroversion, independence, objectivity, originality, personal integrity, resourcefulness, self-confidence, and tolerance of stress.
- Task-related characteristics: Includes the need for achievement, drive for responsibility, enterprise and initiative, responsibility in pursuit of objectives, and task orientation.
- Social characteristics: Includes the ability to enlist cooperation, administrative ability, attractiveness, cooperativeness, nurturance, prestige, sociability and interpersonal skills, social participation, and tact and diplomacy (**TABLE 4-1**).

Stogdill noted that there is no universal set of leader traits that are common across all situational contexts. Stogdill asserted that this does not mean that leader qualities are irrelevant and that scholars ought to focus exclusively on aspects of the situation in the study of leadership. Looking at characteristics of the leader is important in understanding how work units and organizations achieve goals.

More recently, Kirkpatrick and Locke (1991) offered another set of the qualities common among leaders:

- Drive
- Leadership motivation
- Honesty and integrity
- Self-confidence
- Cognitive ability
- Knowledge of task (business)

For Kirkpatrick and Locke, "drive" refers to a general category of important traits that include a high achieve-

Table 4-1 Stogdill 1974 Findings

Intelligence and ability	Intelligence	Judgment and decisiveness	Knowledge
	Fluency of speech		
Personality	Adjustment	Aggressiveness and assertiveness	Alertness
	Ascendance	Emotional balance	Enthusiasm
	Extroversion	Independence	Objectivity
	Originality	Personal integrity	Resourcefulness
	Self-confidence	Tolerance of stress	
Task-related characteristics	Need for achievement	Drive for responsibility	Enterprise and initiative
	Responsible in pursuit of objectives	Task orientation	
Social characteristics	Ability to enlist cooperation	Administrative ability	Attractiveness
	Cooperativeness	Nurturance	Prestige
	Sociability and interpersonal skills	Social participation	Tact and diplomacy

Source: Adapted from Stogdill (1974).

ment motive, ambition, energy, and tenacity. They describe leaders as those who can sustain the needed energy over long periods of time to persevere toward career or work goals. "Leadership motivation" refers to the desire to influence others, which is sometimes known as a "need for power." The desire for power is motivated by two different types of dominance: personalized power motive and socialized power motive. Personalized power motive seeks power as an end in and of itself and focuses on power solely for the sake of dominating others. Socialized power motive, by contrast, is more altruistic in that power is used to achieve desired goals or vision. "Honesty and integrity" are important virtues for all individuals but play a critical role for leaders. Honesty refers to being truthful and nondeceitful, whereas integrity is the connection between words and actions.

"Self-confidence" is an important element in gaining the trust of others. Often there is a close correspondence between self-confidence and other characteristics, such as assertiveness and decisiveness, which can help garner the confidence of others. "Cognitive ability" describes the ability to gather, integrate, and interpret large amounts of information. Cognitive ability is manifested as the capacity to think strategically and multidimensionally. Closely related to cognitive ability is the high degree of "knowledge of the task (business)." Effective leaders gather information about the task, the organization, and the industry. In-depth information helps leaders make effective and well-informed decisions.

Leadership Points to Ponder

Similar in some ways to "Great Man" theories, trait theory assumes that people inherit certain qualities and traits that make them better suited to leadership. Trait theories often identify particular personality or behavioral characteristics shared by leaders. If particular traits are key features of leadership, how does one explain people who possess those qualities but are not leaders? This question is one of the difficulties in using trait theories to explain leadership.

PERSONALITY AND LEADERSHIP

Research has shown over time that personality traits generally comprise five dimensions, also known as the "Big Five" (Digman, 1990; Norman, 1963; **TABLE 4-2**): (1) neuroticism and emotional stability, (2) extraversion and intraversion, (3) openness, (4) agreeableness, and (5) conscientiousness. The five dimensions are relatively independent of one another, and research indicates that they have important implications for organizational performance and leadership.

Research regarding the Big Five personality dimensions has indicated that they are related to various organizational or work outcomes. For instance, Barrick and Mount (1991) analyzed 117 published studies of personality and organizational outcomes. Their meta-analytic study reported that "conscientiousness" was most strongly related to work tasks in all jobs. Put differently, those who were achievement-oriented, dependable, hardworking, and persistent were likely to perform well at their jobs. "Extraversion" was the second strongest correlation to job performance and was especially important for managers and sales personnel. This is not surprising, because both occupations require a high level of social interaction. However, extraversion is not an essential trait for every job at every level in organization. "Openness to experience" was the third most important predictor of job performance. Individuals possessing a high level of openness to experience are typically eager to learn and likely to benefit from training experiences. "Emotional stability" was related to job performance, but the strength of the correlation was relatively low. It is speculated that the relationship between emotional stability and job performance is not a linear, but rather a curvilinear, relationship. This may mean that individuals with a moderate level of anxiety can spur themselves on to succeed. "Agreeableness" was the weakest predictor of job performance, which suggests that being courteous, trusting, and soft-hearted was less important than being talkative, social, and assertive (i.e., extraverted). Although some research has established relationships between personality dimensions and job performance, other research has established more direct linkages between personality and leadership.

Judge, Bono, Ilies, and Gerhardt (2002) analyzed 78 studies that examined the Big Five personality dimensions against leadership emergence and leadership effectiveness. "Leadership emergence" refers to whether (or to what degree) an individual is perceived by others, who have limited information about the individual's actual performance, as a leader. "Leadership effectiveness" describes a leader's performance in influencing activities of his or her unit in achieving its goals (based on Lord, De Vader, & Alliger, 1986). Extraversion was the most important correlate of the Big Five dimensions to both leadership emergence and leadership effectiveness (Judge et al., 2002). Conscientiousness was the second strongest predictor of leadership. Like extraversion, conscientiousness was more strongly linked to leader emergence than leader effectiveness. Openness to experience was related to both leader emergence and leader effectiveness. There was a limited relationship between emotional stability and leader emergence and effectiveness, and agreeableness was the least relevant of the five dimensions.

Table 4-2 Big Five Personality Dimensions

Neuroticism and emotional stability	The degree to which an individual is anxious, nervous, depressed, and insecure
Extraversion and introversion	The tendency of being sociable, talkative, assertive, and having positive energy
Openness	The degree to which an individual is imaginative, creative, curious, and seeking of new experiences
Agreeableness	The degree to which one is accepting, conforming, courteous, good-natured, and nurturing
Conscientiousness	The tendency of being thorough, organized, responsible, and dependable

EMOTIONAL INTELLIGENCE

Salovey and Mayer (1990) originally coined the term "emotional intelligence," which describes aspects of social and interpersonal intelligence. Emotional intelligence largely has to do with the ability to understand one's own and others' emotions and how those emotions affect social relationships. Goldman (1995, 1998) noted that emotional intelligence is comprised of a set of competencies: self-awareness, self-regulation, self-motivation, empathy for others, and interpersonal and social skills (**TABLE 4-3**).

Emotional intelligence has emerged as an important area of psychology and has been emerging as a construct in the field of leadership studies. Researchers found relationships between emotional intelligence and organizational outcomes. For instance, Wong and Law (2002) reported a strong relationship between emotional intelligence and job satisfaction. Furthermore, they found a relationship between leaders' emotional intelligence and their followers' job satisfaction and extra-role behavior; however, there was no direct relationship to followers' job performance.

Leadership Points to Ponder

It is very important to understand that emotional intelligence is not the opposite of intelligence; it is not the triumph of heart over head—it is the unique intersection of both.

David Caruso (from *http://www.6seconds.org*)

Van Rooy and Viswesvaran (2004) reviewed 69 independent studies linking emotional intelligence to performance outcomes. Their study indicated that emotional intelligence was a valuable predictor of performance. Additionally, they reported that emotional intelligence was highly related to the Big Five personality dimensions. This means that there may not be very clear distinctions between personality and emotional intelligence.

Research has also investigated individual components of emotional intelligence. For example, Wolff, Pescosolido, and Druskat (2002) reported that empathic skills play a role in leadership emergence in self-managing teams. This is likely because emergent leaders must understand and coordinate team members without access to and administration of formal rewards and punishments.

George (2000) described how emotions are an important part of leadership. She argued that emotional intelligence is related to leadership in five essential ways

1. Developing a sense of collective goals and objectives
2. Instilling in others the knowledge and appreciation of the importance of work
3. Generating excitement, enthusiasm, confidence, and trust
4. Encouraging flexibility in decision making and change processes
5. Establishing and maintaining a meaningful identify for the organization

There is still debate on the importance of emotional intelligence as it relates to leadership (Antonakis, Ashkanasy, & Dasborough, 2009). Although several studies link aspects of emotional intelligence to leadership (e.g.,

---

Table 4-3 Aspects of Emotional Intelligence

Self-awareness	Being aware of feelings as they happen; the ability to monitor feelings from moment to moment
Self-regulation	The ability to soothe oneself, or to shake off anxiety or irritability
Self-motivation	The capacity to marshal emotions to achieve a goal; remaining positive and optimistic
Empathy for others	Being attuned to social signals that indicate what others want or need; being able to put oneself in their shoes
Interpersonal and social skills	The ability to build and maintain positive relationships with others

Wolff et al., 2002), there is limited empirical research that supports this connection. Furthermore, there is debate about whether emotional intelligence is a broad "trait" definition (e.g., Goldman, 1995) or more a set of abilities (e.g., Salovey & Mayer, 1990).

Emotional intelligence seems to be an important component of leadership. It is reasonable to assume that leaders who are more sensitive to their emotions and the impact of their emotions on others are more effective (Northouse, 2010). More research is needed, however, to understand the intricacies of the relationship between emotional intelligence and leadership.

THE TRAIT APPROACH
Strengths

There are several important strengths of the trait approach to leadership. First, it is intuitively appealing (Northouse, 2010) because it is built on the premise that leaders are somehow different and that the difference rests on special traits that the leader may possess. Leaders are commonly seen as those who are "out in front" of organizations or social movements.

As such, the trait approach provides benchmarks for evaluating what one needs to look for in leaders. For instance, personality assessments can offer valuable insight into individuals' strengths and limitations. Personal assessments can be useful to enhance an individual's overall leadership effectiveness. Additionally, these personal assessments can aid organizations in recruiting, hiring, and training individuals based on particular qualities and abilities.

Weaknesses and Limitations

There are several important limitations of the trait approach to leadership. First, although the trait approach highlights the importance of certain attributes in leaders, it does not explain the leadership process. Leadership is commonly viewed as comprising leaders, followers, and the situation. The trait approach focuses almost exclusively on the leader.

Trait research has consistently failed to establish a universal list of traits that are essential across all situations. Northouse (2010) noted that the list of leader traits seems almost endless. Research has indicated that individuals with a certain trait profile may be effective in

some situations, but ineffective in others. Clearly, leadership requires consideration of other aspects (e.g., followers and situation).

Furthermore, the trait approach has been criticized for the tenuous link between leader traits and outcome variables (e.g., follower performance, organizational performance, satisfaction, and effectiveness). Research has not established a clear understanding of how the qualities of the leader affect group processes and their work.

Finally, the trait approach provides limited insight for training and development. Traits are relatively unchangeable. Therefore, even if research identified a universal set of traits effective across situations, it would be very difficult to help individuals develop those attributes.

LEADER BEHAVIORS
Ohio State Studies

Some of the first research to investigate behaviors of effective leaders occurred in the 1950s. The early research was greatly influenced by studies conducted at Ohio State University. Leadership was defined as "the behavior of an individual when he is directing the activities of a group toward a shared goal" (Hemphill & Coons, 1957, p. 7). This definition informed the development of a comprehensive survey of leader behaviors, the Leader Behavior Description Questionnaire, which was administered to military and civilian personnel (e.g., Halpin & Winer, 1957; Hemphill & Coons, 1957).

Researchers found that leader behavior typically aligned to two broad, independent categories: consideration and initiating structure. "Consideration" refers to behaviors that involve a concern for people and interpersonal relationships. Examples include "looks out for the welfare of team members," "does little things to make it pleasant," and "finds time to listen to team members." "Initiating structure" describes behaviors that demonstrate a concern for task accomplishment. Examples of this category of behaviors include "encourages the use of procedures," "makes performance clear to the team," and "assigns team members particular tasks." Both consideration and initiating structure are independent dimensions of leader behavior. Put differently, managers can demonstrate a high level of consideration while emphasizing a low level of task-related behaviors, or a low level of consideration while displaying a high level of structure. The level to which a leader demonstrates one behavior is not related to the other.

Early research regarding the Leader Behavior Description Questionnaire found that leaders demonstrating high levels of initiating structure experienced greater turnover in their departments than leaders displaying a low level of initiating structure (Fleishman & Harris, 1962). Leaders exhibiting a high degree of consideration experienced less turnover and fewer grievances than those who showed low consideration. This research further revealed that supervisors who demonstrate a high level of consideration could also demonstrate a high level of structure behaviors without a substantial increase in employee grievances.

A meta-analysis technique is one whereby scholars systematically review many studies published on a particular topic. This type of analysis has been conducted on initiating structure and consideration behaviors (e.g., Fisher & Edwards, 1988; Judge, Piccolo, & Ilies, 2004). In general, consideration was positively related to employees' satisfaction with their supervisors, intrinsic job satisfaction, and overall job satisfaction. Fisher and Edwards supported Fleishman's (1972) contention that a leadership style that combines high consideration and high initiating structure will more likely result in leader effectiveness. However, consideration was more closely associated with leader effectiveness than initiating structure. A more recent study extended this support (Judge et al., 2002). Consideration was more strongly related to follower satisfaction with job and satisfaction with leader. Initiating structure was more strongly related to group and organization performance.

Leadership Points to Ponder

If more managers knew about leadership—real leadership, rather than the dribs and drabs of misinformation we all pick up—the world of work would be a much more humane place. What's more, employees would be happier, more engaged, and more productive.

James Manktelow, CEO, MindTools.com

Managerial (Leadership) Grid

Extensive research had been conducted on task-oriented and relationship-oriented leader behaviors. Blake and Mouton (1964, 1978) proposed the managerial grid (**Figure 4-1**), which describes managers in terms of concern for people and concern for production. These general categories of leader behavior parallel the definitions of consideration and initiating structure. Concern for production includes such aspects as quality of policy decisions, efficiency measures, or number of sales or some other physical output. Concern for people refers to activities that display personal commitment, trust, and worth of the individual, and activities that establish good working conditions and interpersonal relationships.

The grid brings together concern for production and concern for people at two intersecting axes. The vertical axis represents concern for people, whereas the horizontal axis represents concern for results. A scale from 1 to 9 runs along each axis: 1 represents low level of concern and 9 represents a high level of concern. Plotting the scores reveals five general combinations of leader behavior: authority-obedience (9,1); country club management (1,9); impoverished management (1,1); middle-of-the-road management (5,5); and team management (9,9).

Authority-Obedience (9,1)

The lower right-hand corner of the grid represents a high concern for results and a low concern for people. This type of leader feels the responsibility to plan and direct the actions of employees to achieve production objectives. This category of leadership is sometime referred to as "management by objectives," which focuses on quotas and deadlines as a means of productivity. Employee reactions to authority-compliance leaders range from resistance to outright resentment.

Country Club Management (1,9)

The upper left corner of the grid is characterized by leaders who give the utmost concern for employees' attitudes and feelings. In this "country club" atmosphere, people essentially do what they enjoy, at their own pace, and with whom they like. Togetherness is the key concept as the leader seeks to create a "one big happy family" environment. With this approach, employees are helped to create goals that they can embrace. Some employees may enjoy the warm and friendly atmosphere, whereas

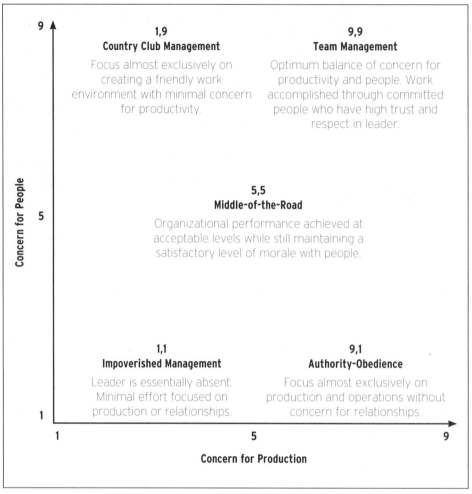

Adapted from Blake & Mouton (1964).

Figure 4-1 Managerial (leadership) grid.

others may feel stifled and unchallenged and, as a result, may become exceedingly frustrated.

Impoverished Management (1,1)

The lower left-hand corner represents a low concern for both people and production. This type of leader has essentially "emotionally resigned and retreated into indifference" (Blake & Mouton, 1978, p. 58). The primary motivation of these individuals is to "go through the motions" and do just enough to preserve their jobs. Typically, the impoverished manager rationalizes the lack of productivity by blaming others or the situation. Managers of this type do not put enough thought into what they might be able to accomplish. Some employees may react to this management style by "going all out" to get recognized and rewarded for the extra effort, seeking to fill the achievement void and thereby advance their careers. Others may find the situation unsatisfactory and transfer within the organization or leave for other opportunities. Some, unfortunately, may follow their leader's example and do the minimum to get by in the job.

Middle-of-the-Road Management (5,5)

Middle-of-the-road managers walk a delicate tightrope in trying to balance the desire to "look good . . . and be 'in' with colleagues" (Blake & Mouton, 1978, p. 75). These managers tend to have superficial convictions because they try to do things that are popular. As a result, they may sacrifice long-term gain for short-term convenience. This approach is "responsive leadership" in that they seek to stay within the bounds of appropriateness and only gradually implement changes within the organization. Some employees may react to this management style by performing in a similar manner, moving along at a steady pace that does not do much to disrupt the status quo. Others may have a more negative reaction because, although they want to contribute more, their efforts go unnoticed, unrecognized, and unappreciated.

Team Management (9,9)

This style of leadership includes a high concern for productivity and people. Effective leaders simultaneously seek opportunities to integrate both personal and corporate goals and objectives. These are achieved through active involvement and participation, which enlists employee commitment to standards of excellence while sustaining full and rewarding experiences. Direction and control are accomplished by helping employees understand problems and their stake in the outcome. Many employees react to this approach with enthusiasm because it fosters involvement and commitment. However, some employees may feel overwhelmed because they are unprepared for the level of participation necessary to successfully operate within this paradigm.

Michigan Studies

A program at the University of Michigan also conducted studies examining leader behaviors around the same time as the Ohio State studies. The Michigan studies looked at the relationship between leader behavior and group processes and also sought to measure group performance. The initial research was conducted via field studies (e.g., Katz & Kahn, 1952; Katz, Maccoby, & Morse, 1950), but a more detailed comparison of leader behaviors was explained more fully by Likert (1961, 1967).

These studies reported three general categories of leader behavior: (1) task-oriented, (2) relations-oriented, and (3) participative leadership. Task-oriented leaders helped work groups achieve performance outcomes, such as coordinating activities, providing necessary supplies, and guiding employees to setting and achieving performance goals. Relations-oriented behaviors aimed to create and maintain appropriate workplace relationships, such as showing of trust and confidence in employees, acting friendly, showing appreciation, and helping employees with career goals. According to Likert,

managers should treat employees in a manner that enhances their sense of self-worth and personal importance. Participative leaders used more group supervision rather than supervising employees independently. Such leaders often made use of group meetings to facilitate communication, cooperation, and group decision making and to resolve conflict among group members.

Unlike the Ohio State studies that reported leader behavior (consideration and initiating structure) along two independent dimensions, the Michigan studies described leader behaviors as operating along a single continuum. Although leaders may demonstrate behaviors consistent with the three general categories identified previously, Likert (1961, 1967) described in detail four systems of organizational and performance characteristics. These systems yield a spectrum of productivity results, from mediocre to excellent (**TABLE 4-4**).

> ### Leadership Points to Ponder
>
> *Leadership should be more participative than directive, more enabling than performing.*
>
> Mary D. Poole (from *http://www.heartquotes.net*)

System I: Exploitive Authoritative

In the exploitive authoritative system, employees are motivated primarily out of fear of negative consequences or punishments. Rarely are they provided with positive rewards. As a result, employees take a subservient and even hostile attitude toward their supervisors. Control in this type of system is concentrated at the top. High performance goals are pressed by the top levels of the organization but are often resisted by employees, which results in mediocre productivity.

System II: Benevolent Authoritative

The benevolent authoritative system is still characterized by motivating employees primarily with negative consequences, but there are more opportunities for positive rewards. Communication is primarily downward through formal channels. Communication that does flow upward is limited and typically filtered information. Employees feel limited responsibility for initiating upward communication. There is high concern for goals at the top of the organization, but some responsibility for goal setting is delegated to middle levels of the organization, which results in fair levels of productivity.

Table 4-4 Organizational and Performance Characteristics of Different Leadership Systems

Operating Characteristics	Exploitive Authoritative	Benevolent Authoritative	Consultative	Participative
Character of motivational forces	Fear, threats, punishment, and occasional rewards	Rewards and some actual or potential punishment	Rewards, occasional punishment, and some involvement	Economic rewards based on compensation system developed through participation; group participation and involvement in setting goals, improving methods, appraising progress toward goals, and so forth
Attitudes toward others	Subservient attitudes toward supervisors	Subservient attitudes toward supervisors; competition for status	Cooperative, reasonably favorable attitudes toward others	Favorable, cooperative attitudes throughout organization
Communication processes	Very little interaction, downward	Little interaction, mostly downward communication	Quite a bit of interaction, communication both upward and downward	High interaction, communication flows easy up, down, and with peers
Character of decision-making processes	Bulk of decisions at top of organization	Policy at the top, many decisions within prescribed framework made at lower levels	Broad policy and general decisions at the top, specific decisions made at lower levels	Decision making widely done throughout organization
Character of goal setting	Orders issued	Orders issued, but opportunity for comment	Goals are set after discussion with employees of problems and actions planned	Typically, goals are established through group participation
Performance characteristics	Mediocre productivity	Fair to good productivity	Good productivity	Excellent productivity

Source: Adapted from Likert (1961).

System III: Consultative

The consultative system focuses more on positive rewards but still maintains negative punishments as motivating factors. Employees are cooperative and typically have favorable attitudes toward others in the organization. Improved communication results in communication channels that flow upward and downward. A moderate amount of teamwork and cooperation, whereby work groups can influence departmental goals, increases employee acceptance of work goals. As a result, this system is characterized by good productivity.

System IV: Participative

The participative system provides employees with extensive opportunities to set goals, appraise progress, and create positive reward opportunities through effective compensation systems. Employees possess highly favorable attitudes toward the organization and have high levels of trust and confidence. Communication flows effectively not only up and down organizational structures, but also with peers across the organization. Considerable responsibility is felt even at the lower levels of the organization. Employees contribute substantially through cooperative decision-making processes, which greatly increases acceptance of work goals. This system is characterized by excellent levels of productivity.

LEADER BEHAVIOR THEORY

Strengths

Leader behavior theory offers several important contributions to the overall understanding of leadership. First, the early leader behavior approach was a major shift in leadership research, which focused almost exclusively on traits of leaders (Northouse, 2010). The focus on leader behaviors emphasized what leaders did rather than the personalities of leaders. Second, there is an impressive body of research regarding leader behaviors, giving credibility to the basic principles of this theory (Northouse, 2010). The Ohio State studies and subsequent research provide ample support for two general categories (task and relationship) of leader behavior.

The underlying tenets of this theory have essentially provided the foundation for many other leadership theories that have emerged in the past six decades. Effective leadership is concerned with both the tasks to be accomplished and the relationships of those participating in the leadership process. The importance of task-oriented and relationship-oriented behaviors cannot be understated.

Limitations and Challenges

The leader behavior approach is not without its limitations. First, research does not adequately explain how exactly the behavior of leaders directly causes important organizational or performance outcomes (Bryman, 1992; Yukl, 2010). Much of the research regarding leader behaviors has been conducted via field studies that measure behaviors by questionnaire. Although these studies can produce useful insights regarding managers' behaviors and organizational outcomes, scholars can only assert that there is a correlation between the variables. This research method cannot assert causality. Researchers using this type of method cannot account for all of the extraneous variables that might influence the connection between leader behaviors and outcomes. Additionally, as with the limitations of the trait perspective of leadership, the behavior approach has not produced a universal set of behaviors that are effective in all situations (Northouse, 2010).

INFLUENCE TACTICS

Influence has long been regarded as an important part of the leadership process. Leadership effectiveness relies on leaders influencing followers and followers influencing leaders. Influence refers to the "change in a target agent's attitudes, values, beliefs or behaviors as a result of influence tactics." Influence tactics refers to an individual's "actual behaviors aimed at changing another person's attitudes, values, beliefs or behaviors" (Hughes, Ginnett, & Curphy, 2005, p. 108).

> ### Leadership Points to Ponder
>
> *There is a secret pride in every human heart that revolts at tyranny. You may order and drive an individual, but you cannot make him respect you.*
>
> William Hazlitt (from *http://www.brainyquote.com*)

Kipnis, Schmidt, and Wilkinson (1980) developed ground-breaking research into organizational influence and developed the original taxonomy of influence tactics. Their research subjects described both successful and unsuccessful influence attempts. Their research revealed eight dimensions of influence:

1. Assertiveness: Includes demanding, ordering, and setting deadlines.
2. Ingratiation: "Acting humble" and "making the other person feel important."
3. Rationality: Using logic and explaining the reason for the request.
4. Sanctions: Includes such behaviors as "preventing salary increases" or "threatening job security."
5. Exchange of benefits: Reminding the target of past favors or personal sacrifices.
6. Upward appeal: Making formal requests to higher levels in the organization and enlisting the support of higher-ups.
7. Blocking: Includes the threat of slowing down work or stopping work with the target.
8. Coalition: Obtaining support of coworkers to apply pressure on the target to comply.

The Profiles of Organizational Influence Strategies survey was developed based on this research (Kipnis & Schmidt, 1982). Numerous studies have used the Profiles of Organizational Influence Strategies and even the revised versions of the survey (e.g., Ansari & Kapoor, 1987), but there has been limited support for the questionnaire as an effective measure of the taxonomy of influence tactics (Hochwarter, Pearson, Ferris, Perrew, & Ralston, 2000).

Yukl and colleagues (Yukl & Falbe, 1990; Yukl, Kim, Perrewe & Falbe, 1996) refined and extended the influence tactics taxonomy. They identified 11 proactive influence tactics

1. Rational persuasion
2. Apprising
3. Inspirational appeal
4. Consultation
5. Exchange
6. Collaboration
7. Personal appeals
8. Ingratiation
9. Legitimating
10. Pressure
11. Coalition

A summary list and definitions are provided in **TABLE 4-5**. Their studies have resulted in the development of the Influence Behavior Questionnaire, which was designed to provide multisource feedback to managers (Yukl, Lepsinger, & Lucia, 1992).

Rational Persuasion

Rational persuasion involves the use of logical arguments and factual information with the aim of influencing the target. Strong forms of rational persuasion involve

Table 4-5 Definition of Influence Tactics Measured by the Influence Behavior Questionnaire (IBQ and IBQ-G)

Tactic	Definition
Rational persuasion	The person uses logical arguments and factual evidence to persuade you that a proposal or request is viable and likely to result in the attainment of task objectives.
Apprising	The person points out how the request will personally benefit you. *Added in Yukl, Chavez, & Seifert (2005)*
Inspirational appeal	The person makes an emotional request or proposal that arouses enthusiasm by appealing to your values and ideals or by increasing your confidence that you can do it.
Consultation	The person persuades you and others to suggest improvements or recommendations to enlist your support for the change or activity.
Exchange	The person makes an explicit or implicit promise that you will receive rewards or tangible benefits if you comply with a request or support a proposal, or reminds you of a prior favor to be reciprocated.
Collaboration	The person offers assistance and resources if you carry out the request. *Added in Yukl, Chavez, & Seifert (2005)*
Personal appeal	The person makes a request by appealing to your friendship or personal loyalty or by requesting a personal favor.
Ingratiation	The person seeks to get you in a good mood or to think favorably of him or her before asking you to do something.
Legitimating	The person makes a request by appealing to your authority or citing relevant rules or policies.
Pressure	The person uses demands, threats, or intimidation to convince you to comply with a request or to support a proposal.
Coalition	The person seeks the aid of others to persuade you to do something or uses the support of others as an argument for you to agree also.

Source: Yukl & Falbe (1990); Yukl, Chavez, & Seifert (2005).

detailed explanations of the reasons for proposals and their importance and can also include logical inferences and opinions based on factual information (Yukl, 2010). This tactic is used in all directions in organizational hierarchy: upward, downward, and laterally. However, research indicates that it is more commonly used to influence targets upward in the organization (Yukl, Falbe, & Youn, 1993; Yukl & Tracey, 1990).

The use of rational persuasion has positive outcomes. For instance, compared to ineffective managers, effective managers more frequently use rational persuasion (Yukl, Seifert, & Chavez, 2008). Additionally research indicates that individuals who use rationality are more likely to experience extrinsic success, such as success in their careers (Higgins, Judge, & Ferris, 2003).

Inspirational Appeal

Inspirational appeal involves an emotional, values-based appeal aimed at arousing target enthusiasm. This contrasts with rational persuasion, which develops logical arguments, in that it seeks to link to the target person's values, hopes, or ideals. Some values may include fairness, justice, liberty, equality, love, excellence, and humanitarianism (Yukl, 2010).

Inspirational appeal is used regardless of direction in the organization: upward, downward, or lateral (Yukl et al., 1996; Yukl et al., 2008; Yukl & Tracey, 1990). However, it is more commonly used in a downward direction from managers to their direct reports and laterally between peers in organizations (Falbe & Yukl, 1992).

Effective managers more commonly use inspirational appeals, compared to ineffective managers (Yukl et al., 2008). However the quality of the manager–direct report relationship seems to affect the tactic's effectiveness. For instance, when there was a low-quality relationship, the use of inspirational appeals by the manager was negatively related to direct report helping behavior (Sparrowe, Soetjipto, & Kraimer, 2006). Put differently, employees who have a poor relationship with their managers perceived the appeal to values as being hollow and were not willing to exert extra-role behavior.

Consultation

Consultation invites the target to participate and offer suggestions in carrying out an initiative or proposed change. The primary purpose of the tactic is to foster the target's support for a decision already made by the agent (Yukl, 2010). Consultation is widely considered an effective influence tactic that results in target commitment regardless of directional use in the organization (Yukl & Falbe, 1990; Yukl & Tracey, 1990) but is more commonly used in a downward or lateral direction (Falbe & Yukl, 1992). Employees who perceive their managers as effective reported that their managers frequently make use of consultation techniques (Yukl et al., 2008).

Pressure

Pressure occurs when an agent uses threats, warnings, or other assertive behavior such as repeated checking to see if the target has complied with the request. Pressure tactics may produce compliance with a particular request, but research also suggests that its use may result in resistance more than compliance or commitment (Yukl et al., 1996). Pressure tactics are negatively related to commitment from direct reports or peers (Yukl et al., 2008; Yukl & Tracey, 1990).

Pressure is most commonly used in a downward direction in organizational structures (e.g., from managers to their direct reports; Yukl & Tracey, 1990). However, managers who make frequent use of pressure tactics are perceived as being ineffective (Yukl et al., 2008). Therefore, pressure is considered an ineffective influence tactic.

Ingratiation

Ingratiation involves the use of praise or flattery to make the target feel better about himself or herself before the request. This may involve the giving of compliments, doing unsolicited favors, or acting particularly friendly. This approach is more commonly used in a lateral or downward direction in organizational hierarchies (Yukl et al., 1993) and can result in a mixture of compliance and commitment (Yukl & Falbe, 1990; Yukl & Tracey, 1990).

The quality of the manager–direct report relationship affects the effectiveness of this tactic. Furst and Cable (2008) found that when the relationship between managers and direct reports is poor, direct reports are more likely to resist the influence attempt. This suggests that employees accustomed to an antagonistic relationship with their managers are likely to view the influence attempt with suspicion and therefore resist.

Exchange

Exchange involves the implicit or explicit offering of some future benefits that the target perceives as meaningful in return for carrying out a particular request. Exchange attempts are a way to increase the benefits to make it worthwhile for the target to fulfill a particular request. It is more common for exchange tactics to be used in a lateral and downward direction in organizational hierarchies, and research has also indicated that it can result in target commitment from peers and subordinates (Yukl et al., 1993; Yukl & Tracey, 1990). It is used less to influence in the upward direction in organizations.

The quality of the manager–direct report relationship affects the effectiveness of exchange tactics. For instance, low-quality manager–direct report relationships are negatively related to employee helping behavior (Sparrowe et al., 2006). This indicates that employees view the exchange as empty and are therefore unwilling to fulfill requests beyond normal job responsibilities.

Coalition

Coalition occurs when the agent of the influence attempt seeks help from other people to influence the target person. The coalition of partners can come from a variety of sources including peers, subordinates, superiors, or outsiders. This style of influence is successful if the target respects or likes the individuals in the coalition.

Coalition is more likely to be used to influence peers or superiors (Yukl et al., 1993; Yukl & Tracey, 1990). It is generally perceived as an ineffective tactic (Yukl & Tracey, 1990) that results more commonly in resistance or compliance rather than commitment (Falbe & Yukl, 1992). Usually, it is only effective to enlist support for an organizational change rather than to help an employee work faster or to improve performance.

Legitimating

Legitimating seeks to establish an individual's authority or right to make a request. Legitimating tactics include an appeal to organizational hierarchy or norms or other organizational policies. This style of influence is more commonly used in a downward or lateral direction (Yukl et al., 1993). Legitimating may result in compliance or resistance (Falbe & Yukl, 1992), but research indicates that it is negatively related to target commitment (Yukl & Tracey, 1990). The quality of the manager–direct report

relationship can affect the effectiveness of this tactic. In manager–direct report relationships that are characterized by antagonism, legitimating tactics result in greater resistance from employees (Furst & Cable, 2008).

Personal Appeal

Personal appeal refers to asking someone to do a favor out of friendship or loyalty. By its very nature, the style is not effective if used when the target person dislikes the agent making the request. However, the stronger the relationship, the more latitude the agent has to make a request based on a personal appeal (Yukl, 2010).

Personal appeals are more common in a lateral direction (Yukl et al., 1993); however, the tactic can result in commitment from peers and subordinates (Yukl & Tracey, 1990). This approach can result in a mixture of commitment and compliance and is perceived as a moderately effective influence tactic (Falbe & Yukl, 1992).

Collaboration and Apprising

Two new influence tactics have recently been identified: collaboration and apprising (Yukl, Chavez, & Seifert, 2005). Collaboration refers to the offering of necessary resources or assistance if the target will carry out the request. These requests may involve showing the target how to perform a task or deal with a problem, or may involve providing necessary equipment for a task. Collaboration is different from exchange tactics in that exchanges typically involve impersonal benefits (Yukl, 2010). Collaboration, however, involves joint effort to accomplish an objective.

Apprising occurs when the agent of the request explains how a request will benefit the target personally. For instance, a manager may explain how a request will be an opportunity for individuals to develop new skills necessary for their careers. Unlike exchanges, the benefits for the target person are the by-product of the task itself rather than something provided directly by the agent (Yukl, 2010).

Both collaboration and apprising influence tactics are comparatively new and have not been extensively researched. Initial research has indicated that both collaboration and apprising are positively related to target commitment (Yukl et al., 2008); however, more research is required to understand the nature of their use and overall effectiveness.

TABLE **4-6** identifies general research trends regarding the directional use of each of the influence tactics and the typical level of effectiveness.

Strengths

The theory of influence tactics offers several important advantages over prior research regarding leadership. First, the development of taxonomies and subsequent research on influence tactics offers more specific categories of behavior compared to the meta-categories of task- and relationship-oriented leadership styles. In addition, research in this area has attempted to explain the likely target response of the influence attempt (e.g., commitment, compliance, or resistance) among other outcome variables.

Weaknesses and Limitations

As with other perspectives of leadership, influence tactics theory is not without limitations. One limitation is that research has not been able to establish a universal set of influence tactics that have proved effective across contexts, thus limiting the value of the theory in leadership instruction. In addition, some scholars categorize the influence tactics into the meta-categories of "hard" (e.g., pressure, coalition, legitimating, and exchange) and "soft" (e.g., inspirational appeal, consultation, personal appeal, and ingratiation) tactics (Yukl, 2010). This classification then defeats the purpose of trying to identify and understand specific leader behaviors and how they affect followers or other organizational outcomes.

Third, most of the research regarding influence tactics treats each influence attempt as an isolated episode (Yukl, 2010). An understanding of influence should be considered in the larger context of the overall leadership process whereby there is often a reciprocal influence process between leaders and followers and relationships that evolve over time. Some research has begun to examine the use of influence tactics in combination with each other and the sequencing of tactic use (Yukl et al., 1993). Furthermore, only a few studies have examined influence tactics within the context of the manager–direct report relationship (Furst & Cable, 2008). This helps shed light on why some influence tactics are met with resistance among some targets, whereas other targets respond with compliance or commitment. Additional research is needed to more fully understand the use and

Table 4-6 Summary of Findings for Influence Tactics

Influence Tactic	Directional Use More Frequently	General Effectiveness
Rational persuasion	All directions	High
Apprising	Down than lateral and up	Moderate
Inspirational appeal	Down than up and lateral	High
Consultation	Down and lateral than up	High
Exchange	Down and lateral than up	Moderate
Collaboration	Down and lateral than up	High
Personal appeal	Lateral than down and up	Moderate
Ingratiation	Down and lateral than up	Moderate
Legitimating	Down and lateral than up	Low
Pressure	Down than lateral and up	Low
Coalition	Lateral and up than down	Low/moderate

Source: Yukl, 2010.

effectiveness of influence tactics in the episodic nature of leadership.

CHARISMATIC LEADERSHIP

Recent theories of charismatic leadership were largely influenced by the early work of Max Weber (1947). Charisma derives from the Greek word, also *charisma*, which means a "divinely inspired gift." According to Weber, charisma described the "certain quality of an individual personality by virtue of which he is set apart from ordinary men" (p. 358). Weber described these exceptional qualities as being divine in origin and not accessible to ordinary individuals.

Weber (1947) asserted that leaders who possess charisma have a "duty of those who have been called to a charismatic mission to recognize its quality and to act accordingly" (p. 359). Charismatic influence is outside of formal authority and based largely on follower perceptions of the "divine inspiration." Recognition of the charismatic gift is freely given to the leader because of miracles or other proof of the gift. Charismatic leaders inspire "hero worship" and absolute trust and devotion of followers. The leader's charisma inspires deep-seated enthusiasm and hope in times of social crisis. As a result, charismatic authority can be a tremendous revolutionary force.

In recent decades, numerous scholars have offered versions of charismatic leadership theory, often departing from the Weber's original conceptualization. These neo-charismatic theories of leadership (Conger & Kanungo, 1987; House, 1977) describe leaders' motives and behaviors and the effect they have on followers.

Charismatic Leadership: A Self-Concept Theory

House (1977) examined leadership in terms of the effects of leaders on followers. Leaders who have an unusually high charismatic effect on followers are deemed charis-

matic leaders. These effects are framed in emotional rather than calculative terms. As such, charismatic leaders arouse follower loyalty, commitment, devotion, and enthusiasm. Shamir, House, and Arthur (1993) later clarified and extended this theory and developed testable propositions of charismatic leadership. Followers perceive this type of leader as possessing extremely high levels of self-confidence and strong and correct convictions about the moral righteousness of their beliefs.

Charismatic leaders combine both traits and behaviors to achieve a profound effect on followers. Leader traits include a strong need for power, high self-confidence, high need for social influence, and a strong conviction in their own beliefs. These qualities are then displayed through a variety of behaviors: role modeling, image building, goal articulation, and exhibiting of high expectations. Charismatic leaders are often seen as role models. They display actions that are consistent with a set of core values and beliefs. In turn, followers subscribe to these values and beliefs because it enhances their self-esteem and self-worth. Charismatic leaders demonstrate image-building behaviors intended to create impressions of their own competence and success.

Leaders of this type are also effective communicators because they persuasively articulate "transcendent" goals. These goals are laden with moral overtones because they are more ideologic goals than pragmatic goals. As a result, the leader's vision becomes a shared vision for what the future could be. In addition to persuasively presenting compelling possibilities for the future, charismatic leaders also exhibit high expectations and demonstrate strong confidence in followers. This type of leader influences the kinds of rewards sought by followers and their motivation to perform effectively. The charismatic leader communicates messages that arouse follower motives that are especially relevant in achieving the mission. Weber (1947) asserted that charismatic leaders were born out of a crisis. House (1977) maintained that stressful situations were not a necessary condition for charismatic leadership; however, charismatic leaders can be instrumental in appealing to followers in ideologic terms.

Charismatic Leadership: An Attribution Theory

Conger and Kanungo (1987) developed a theory of charismatic leadership where attributions of charisma are made by followers who observe certain behaviors in a given situation. Attribution of charismatic leadership depends on leader behavior that can be categorized based on three stages of the charismatic leadership process (Conger & Kanugo, 1988; **Figure 4-2**).

The first stage involves an evaluation of the status quo. Charismatic leaders effectively assess environmental resources and constraints. Additionally, they are sensitive to the abilities, needs, and emotions of followers and the context in which they operate. Leaders who are perceived as taking on extraordinarily high personal risks are likely to be attributed with charisma. Risks can include the possible loss of finances, informal status, power, or credibility. Leaders attributed with charisma effectively make use of personal power. "Charismatic personal power stems from the elitist idealized vision, the entrepreneurial advocacy of radical changes, and the depth of knowledge and expertise to help achieve desired objectives" (Conger & Kanungo, 1987, p. 644).

During stage two, charismatic leaders formulate and articulate new organizational goals. According to Conger and Kanungo (1987), leaders play a major role in creating the need for change. Leaders can frame the status quo as unacceptable, which can cause followers to become disenchanted with the present social order and therefore experience psychologic distress. This distress then facilitates a context for the emergence of charismatic leadership. Charisma is likely attributed to leaders who communicate a utopian vision for the future that substantially differs from the status quo. Leaders must present the status quo as something that is negative and intolerable, especially in comparison to the idealized

vision. If the vision is within the latitude of acceptance, followers attribute charisma to the leader.

Within the final stage of the charismatic leadership process, leaders communicate the means by which to achieve the new vision. Leaders attributed with charisma also use innovative, unconventional strategies to achieve the vision. Such strategies are needed to overcome the inertia of maintaining the status quo to actualize the utopian vision. Their appeal to followers includes communicating their own motivation to lead and express, both verbally and nonverbally, the commitment to their convictions and confidence in their abilities to lead.

Stage Model of Charismatic Leadership

Conger (1989) further refined and extended the theory to describe a sequential series of activities (or stages) of charismatic leader behavior. Stage one involves the leader making an assessment of the strategic opportunities and constraints of the environment, both internal and external to the organization. Because organizations are in a constant state of flux, this stage is an ongoing process. Two other critical skills of this stage include sensitivity to constituents' needs and the ability to see untapped opportunities or deficiencies in current situations.

The second stage includes the articulation of an idealized vision. The utopian vision provides employees with a tremendous challenge and motivation for change. The charismatic leader creates a compelling case for how the current situation is unacceptable, while at the same time describing their vision as the most attractive option for the future.

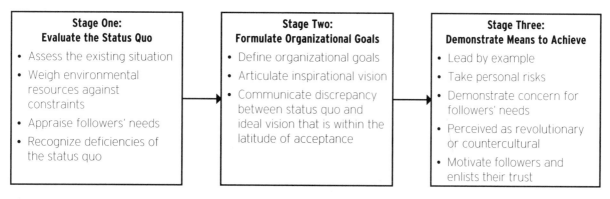

Stage One: Evaluate the Status Quo	Stage Two: Formulate Organizational Goals	Stage Three: Demonstrate Means to Achieve
• Assess the existing situation • Weigh environmental resources against constraints • Appraise followers' needs • Recognize deficiencies of the status quo	• Define organizational goals • Articulate inspirational vision • Communicate discrepancy between status quo and ideal vision that is within the latitude of acceptance	• Lead by example • Take personal risks • Demonstrate concern for followers' needs • Perceived as revolutionary or countercultural • Motivate followers and enlists their trust

Source: Adapted from Conger & Kanungo (1988).

Figure 4-2 Stages of charismatic leadership.

Stage three is characterized by developing follower buy-in to the vision. The leader elicits desire and trust among followers through personal risk-taking, self-sacrifice, and unconventional expertise. In part, leaders are able to achieve extraordinary levels of trust and commitment by showing concern for followers' needs rather than self-interests. Leaders further develop trust by appearing as experts, particularly in the area of using nontraditional methods to achieve organizational goals.

The final stage is accomplishing the vision. Because of their extraordinary use of personal examples, role modeling, and unconventional tactics, charismatic leaders differ from others. Through praise, charismatics instill in followers the belief in their ability to achieve the vision.

Research on Charismatic Leadership

Scholars have studied the nature and effects of charismatic leadership. Conger and Kanungo (1998) developed and refined a survey to measure five dimensions of charismatic leadership

1. Strategic vision and articulation: The ability of the leader to provide an inspirational possibility for the future in an exciting and enthusiastic manner.

2. Sensitivity to the environment: The ability to recognize environmental conditions both internal and external to the organization.

3. Sensitivity to members' needs: The expression of personal concern for the needs and feelings of others in the organization.

4. Personal risk: Behaviors that may incur a high personal cost for the sake of the organization.

5. Unconventional behavior: Unique and nontraditional behaviors directed at achieving organizational objectives.

Although psychometrically sound surveys have been developed to assess the five dimensions of charismatic leader behavior (e.g., the Conger-Kanungo Scale as reported in Conger, Kanungo, Menon, & Mathur, 1997), much of the research has actually examined charismatic leadership as a global construct along a single meta-dimension.

Some of the research on the outcomes of charismatic leadership has produced mixed results. For example, studies have reported a positive relationship between charismatic leadership and employee job satisfaction (e.g., Rowold & Heinitz, 2007); however, others have not confirmed this relationship (e.g., Conger, Kanungo, & Menon, 2000).

DeGroot, Kiker, and Cross (2000) conducted a meta-analysis of 36 studies that examined charismatic leadership. The study reported that charismatic leadership was related to leader effectiveness, employee performance, and employee commitment to the organization. However, it was not related to employee job satisfaction or employee effort.

One study reported on the relationship between the five independent dimensions of the Conger-Kanungo Scale on organizational outcome variables (Conger et al., 2000). Reverence in the leader as perceived by followers was most strongly related to Sensitivity to the Environment but was also related to Strategic Vision and Articulation and Sensitivity to Member Needs. Employee satisfaction is positively related to three of the charismatic leadership dimensions: Strategic Vision and Articulation, Sensitivity to the Environment, and Sensitivity to Member Needs. Collective Identity is achieved largely through the subscales of Vision Articulation and Sensitivity to Member Needs. Group Performance and Empowerment are related to two dimensions of charismatic leadership: Strategic Vision and Sensitivity to the Environment. The use of Unconventional Behaviors was not related to any of the outcome variables in the study. It seems that two of the five dimensions of charismatic leadership are more important in achieving positive organizational outcomes: Strategic Vision and Articulation and Sensitivity to the Environment.

Dark Side of Charisma

A number of theories of charismatic leadership emphasize its positive aspects and consequences. However, scholars have also considered what is commonly described as the "dark side" of charisma (Conger, 1989; Hogan, Raskin, & Fazzini, 1990). Often, the dark side of charisma focuses on the power motives of the leaders. Howell (1988) differentiated between two types of power: personalized and socialized charisma. Socialized leaders focus their efforts on satisfying organizational and follower needs congruent with shared values. However, personalized leaders focus on getting followers to identify with their personal values and ideologic aims. This type of charismatic leader abuses power for self-serving ends.

For instance, they "exaggerate positive achievement and take unwarranted credit . . . cover up mistakes and failures . . . blame others for mistakes . . . and limit communication of criticism and dissent" (Yukl, 1999, p. 296).

Optimism and self-confidence are important qualities of charismatic leaders. However, these strengths can be taken too far. Excessive optimism makes it more difficult for leaders to recognize and identify genuine flaws in the vision and strategy and leads to bad decision making (Yukl, 2010).

Furthermore, charisma can have negative consequences for those who are led. For instance, some individuals may identify too closely with the charismatic leader and thus not be able to objectively evaluate the vision and strategy. Being in awe of the leader reduces others' ability to offer good recommendations to enhance the strategy. Charismatic leaders use unconventional tactics to achieve organizational objectives; these behaviors can antagonize and offend others who consider the behaviors disruptive and inappropriate (Yukl, 2010).

Strengths

There are a number of unique contributions that the study of charismatic leadership has made toward the overall understanding of the leadership process. First, charismatic leadership theory helps one understand how some leaders achieve exceptional influence with others that is not adequately explained by other theories (Yukl, 2010). Another closely related strength is that it emphasizes the emotional reaction of followers to their leaders, whereas other theories focus on more rational or cognitive-oriented perspectives of the leader–follower interaction. Finally, charismatic leadership theory acknowledges the importance of symbolic behaviors and the leader's role in making events meaningful for followers. By effectively articulating a compelling ideologic vision, followers can internalize organizational goals espoused by the leader during periods of considerable anxiety.

Limitations and Challenges

There are several criticisms of charismatic leadership theory. First, and perhaps most importantly, there is a lack of clarity and consistency in the term "charismatic" (Yukl, 1999). Scholars have offered a variety of definitions of charisma that combine different traits and behaviors of leaders, which has led to confusion about the

construct and has hindered research and understanding of the impact of charisma in the leadership process.

A related limitation is the essential behaviors of charisma. Much of the research on charisma has emphasized socially acceptable behaviors (e.g., articulating ideologic vision, demonstrating confidence); however, there has been little emphasis on manipulative behaviors (e.g., covering up mistakes, exaggerating achievements, limiting follower access to information). Further research is required to more fully understand the "dark side" of charismatic leadership.

Additionally, comparatively little emphasis has been placed on the conditions that facilitate the emergence of charismatic leadership. Theories assert that when followers are insecure, the organization is in serious trouble, or members of an organization are experiencing considerable anxiety and panic, then individuals are more likely to attribute charisma to leaders (e.g., Bligh, Kohles, & Meindl, 2004). More emphasis should be placed on understanding the characteristics of followers and other contextual variables as they are related to leader characteristics.

Finally, there is a lack of a connection between charismatic leadership and organizational effectiveness (Yukl, 1999). Charismatic leadership theory asserts that leaders make radical changes in strategy and culture for the organization. There is only limited support for the relationship between charismatic leadership and improved organizational performance (Waldman, Javidan, & Varella, 2004). Further research is required to understand how charismatic leadership, in combination with other internal and external organizational factors, contributes to organizational effectiveness.

Leadership Points to Ponder

Charisma is the result of effective leadership, not the other way around.

Warren Bennis and Burt Nanus,
(from *http://www.leadershipnow.com*)

SUMMARY

This chapter describes some of the early systematic approaches to the study of leadership. Early work in this area sought to describe a universal set of characteristics of leaders that differentiated them from nonleaders. Both of Stogdill's reviews (1948, 1974) identified general traits that seemed to be common; however, there was no consistent set of traits that are considered to be universal across all times and all contexts.

More recent work in the area of trait research describes the emotional intelligence of leaders and the understanding of their own and others' emotions. It is believed that leaders who are highly attuned to their emotions and are sensitive about how their emotions affect others likely help facilitate positive outcomes. More research is required in this area to understand this linkage.

Early behavior research focused primarily on two very broad categories of leader behavior: task-oriented and relationship-oriented behaviors (e.g., the Ohio State studies, the managerial grid). Research has established several connections between these broad categories and work outcomes. More recent research in the area of leader behaviors offers more specific taxonomies of behavior in the form of influence tactics. Like trait theory, behavioral theories of leadership have not produced a consistent pattern of leader behaviors that are effective across all contexts. However, research in this area does suggest that some influence tactics will likely be more effective than others in given situations.

Wrap-Up

ACTIVITY

Emotional Intelligence Exercise

This activity is intended to challenge you to reflect on your own emotional intelligence abilities. Answer the following reflection questions based on your current ability for each of the five dimensions of emotional intelligence.

1. Which of these capacities have you already developed well? Explain.

2. Which of these capacities do you still need to develop further? Explain.

3. Specify what you can do to further develop these capacities during the next 2 weeks.

Aspects of Emotional Intelligence	
Self-awareness	Being aware of feelings as they happen; the ability to monitor feelings from moment to moment
Self-regulation	The ability to soothe oneself or to shake off anxiety or irritability
Self-motivation	The capacity to marshal emotions to achieve a goal; remaining positive and optimistic
Empathy for others	Being attuned to social signals that indicate what others want or need; being able to put oneself in their shoes
Interpersonal and social skills	The ability to build and maintain positive relationships with others

Influence Tactic Exercise

This activity is intended to provide you with an opportunity to reflect on the tactics you commonly use to influence others around you. Take a moment and ask three of your coworkers to respond to the following survey items regarding your influence tactic use. Each item identifies the category and definition of each influence tactic. After having three coworkers complete the survey, reflect on these reflection questions.

Reflection questions for influence tactic activity:

1. Which tactics did your coworkers identify you use the most? Least?
2. Based on the reading, which influence tactics are typically considered highly effective? Least effective?
3. What steps will you take this week to use highly effective influence tactics more frequently?

(0 = Not at all ; 3 = Sometimes used ; 6 = Commonly useful, almost always)							
Rational persuasion: The person uses logical arguments and factual evidence to persuade you that a proposal or request is viable and likely to result in the attainment of task objectives.	0	1	2	3	4	5	6
Apprising: The person points out how the request will personally benefit you.	0	1	2	3	4	5	6
Inspirational appeal: The person makes an emotional request or proposal that arouses enthusiasm by appealing to your values and ideals, or by increasing your confidence that you can do it.	0	1	2	3	4	5	6
Consultation: The person persuades you and others to suggest improvements or recommendations to enlist your support for the change or activity.	0	1	2	3	4	5	6
Exchange: The person makes an explicit or implicit promise that you will receive rewards or tangible benefits if you comply with a request or support a proposal, or reminds you of a prior favor to be reciprocated.	0	1	2	3	4	5	6
Collaboration: The person offers assistance and resources if you carry out the request.	0	1	2	3	4	5	6
Personal appeal: The person makes a request by appealing to your friendship or personal loyalty or by requesting a personal favor.	0	1	2	3	4	5	6
Ingratiation: The person seeks to get you in a good mood or to think favorably of him or her before asking you to do something.	0	1	2	3	4	5	6
Legitimating: The person makes a request by appealing to your authority or citing relevant rules or policies.	0	1	2	3	4	5	6
Pressure: The person uses demands, threats, or intimidation to convince you to comply with a request or to support a proposal.	0	1	2	3	4	5	6
Coalition: The person seeks the aid of others to persuade you to do something or uses the support of others as an argument for you to agree also.	0	1	2	3	4	5	6

REFERENCES

Ansari, M. A., & Kapoor, A. (1987). Organizational context and upward influence tactics. *Organizational Behavior and Human Decision Processes, 40*, 39–40.

Antonakis, J., Ashkanasy, N. M., & Dasborough, M. T. (2009). Does leadership need emotional intelligence? *Leadership Quarterly, 20*, 247–261.

Barrick, M. R., & Mount, M. K. (1991). The Big Five personality dimensions and job performance: A meta-analysis. *Personnel Psychology, 44*(1), 1–26.

Blake, R. R., & Mouton, J. S. (1964). *The managerial grid.* Houston, TX: Gulf Publishing.

Blake, R. R., & Mouton, J. S. (1978). *The new managerial grid.* Houston, TX: Gulf Publishing.

Bligh, M. C., Kohles, J. C., & Meindl, J. R. (2004). Charisma under crisis: Presidential leadership, rhetoric, and media responses before and after the September 11 terrorist attacks. *Leadership Quarterly, 15*(2), 211–240.

Bryman, A. (1992). *Charisma and leadership in organization.* London, UK: Sage.

Carlyle, T. (1907). *Heroes and hero worship.* Boston, MA: Adams.

Conger, J. A. (1989). *The charismatic leader: Behind the mystique of exceptional leadership.* San Francisco, CA: Jossey-Bass.

Conger, J. A., & Kanungo, R. N. (1987). Toward a behavioral theory of charismatic leadership in organizational settings. *Academy of Management Review, 12*(4), 637–647.

Conger, J. A., & Kanungo, R. N. (1988). Behavioral dimensions of charismatic leadership. In J. A. Conger, R. N. Kanungo, & Associates (Eds.), *Charismatic leadership* (pp. 78–97). San Francisco, CA: Jossey-Bass.

Conger, J. A., & Kanungo, R. N. (1998). *Charismatic leadership in organizations.* Thousand Oaks, CA: Sage.

Conger, J. A., Kanungo, R. N., & Menon, S. T. (2000). Charismatic leadership and follower effects. *Journal of Organizational Behavior, 21*, 747–767.

Conger, J. A., Kanungo, R. N., Menon, S. T., & Mathur, P. (1997). Measuring charisma: Dimensionality and validity of the Conger-Kanungo Scale of charismatic leadership. *Canadian Journal of Administrative Sciences, 14*(3), 290–302.

DeGroot, T., Kiker, D. S., & Cross, T. C. (2000). A meta-analysis to review organizational outcomes related to charismatic leadership. *Canadian Journal of Administrative Sciences, 17*(4), 356–371.

Digman, J. M. (1990). Personality structure: Emergence of the five-factor model. *Annual Review of Psychology, 41*, 417–440.

Falbe, C. M., & Yukl, G. (1992). Consequences for managers of using single influence tactics and combinations of tactics. *Academy of Management Journal, 35*(3), 638–652.

Fisher, B. M., & Edwards, J. E. (1988). Consideration and initiating structure and their relationships with leader effectiveness: A meta-analysis. *Academy of Management Review, 10*, 803–813.

Fleishman, E. A. (1972). *Manual for supervisory behavior description questionnaire.* Washington, DC: American Institutes for Research.

Fleishman, E. A., & Harris, E. F. (1962). Patterns of leadership behavior related to employee grievances and turnover. *Personnel Psychology, 15*, 43–56.

Furst, S. A., & Cable, D. M. (2008). Employee resistance to organizational change: Managerial influence tactics and leader-member exchange. *Journal of Applied Psychology, 93*(2), 453–462.

Galton, R. (1869). *Heredity genius.* New York, NY: Appleton.

George, J. M. (2000). Emotions and leadership: The role of emotional intelligence. *Human Relations, 54*, 1027–1055.

Goldman, D. (1995). *Emotional intelligence.* New York, NY: Bantam.

Goldman, D. (1998). *Working with emotional intelligence.* New York, NY: Bantam.

Halpin, A. W., & Winer, B. J. (1957). A factorial study of the leader behavior descriptions. In R. M. Stogdill & A. E. Coons (Eds.), *Leader behavior: Its description and measurement* (pp. 39–51). Columbus: Bureau of Business Research, Ohio State University.

Hemphill, J. K., & Coons, A. E. (1957). Development of the leader behavior description questionnaire. In R. M. Stogdill & A. E. Coons (Eds.), *Leader behavior: Its description and measurement* (pp. 6–38). Columbus: Bureau of Business Research, Ohio State University.

Higgins, C. A., Judge, T. A., & Ferris, G. R. (2003). Influence tactics and work outcomes: A meta-analysis. *Journal of Organizational Behavior, 24,* 89–106.

Hochwarter, W. A., Pearson, A. W., Ferris, G. R., Perrewe, P. A., & Ralston, D. A. (2000). A re-examination of Schriescheim and Hinkin's measure of upward influence. *Educational and Psychological Measurement, 60,* 755–771.

Hogan, R., Raskin, R., & Fazzini, D. (1990). The dark side of charisma. In K. Clark & M. Clark (Eds.), *Measures of leadership* (pp. 343–354). West Orange, NJ: Leadership Library of America.

House, R. (1977). A 1976 theory of charismatic leadership. In J. G. Hunt & L. L. Larson (Eds.), *Leadership: The cutting edge* (pp. 189–207). Carbondale: Southern Illinois University Press.

Howell, J. M. (1988). Two faces of charisma: Socialized and personalized leadership in organization. In J. A. Conger & R. N. Kanungo (Eds.), *Charismatic leadership: The illusive factor in organizational effectiveness* (pp. 213–236). San Francisco, CA: Jossey-Bass.

Hughes, R. L., Ginnett, R. C., & Curphy, G. J. (2005). *Leadership: Enhancing the lessons of experience.* New York, NY: McGraw-Hill.

Judge, T. A., Bono, J. E., Ilies, R., & Gerhardt, M. W. (2002). Personality and leadership: A qualitative and quantitative review. *Journal of Applied Psychology, 87,* 765–780.

Judge, T. A., Piccolo, R. F., & Ilies, R. (2004). The forgotten ones? The validity of consideration and initiating structure in leadership research. *Journal of Applied Psychology, 89*(1), 36–51.

Katz, D., & Kahn, R. L. (1952). Some recent findings in human-relations research in industry: In E. Swanson, T. Newcomb, & E. Hartley (Eds.), *Readings in social psychology* (pp. 650–665). New York, NY: Holt.

Katz, D., Maccoby, N., & Morse, N. (1950). *Productivity, supervision, and morale in an office situation.* Ann Arbor, MI: Institute for Social Research.

Kipnis, D., & Schmidt, S. M. (1982). *Profile of organizational influence strategies.* San Diego, CA: University Associates.

Kipnis, D., Schmidt, S. M., & Wilkinson, I. (1980). Intra-organizational influence tactics: Exploration in getting one's way. *Journal of Applied Psychology, 65*(4), 440–452.

Kirkpatrick, S. A., & Locke, E. A. (1991). Leadership: Do traits matter? *The Academy of Management Executive, 5,* 48–60.

Likert, R. (1961). *New patterns of management.* New York, NY: McGraw-Hill.

Likert, R. (1967). *The human organization: Its management and value.* New York, NY: McGraw-Hill.

Lord, R. G., De Vader, C. L., & Alliger, G. M. (1986). A meta-analysis of the relation between personality traits and leadership perceptions: An application of validity generalization procedures. *Journal of Applied Psychology, 71,* 402–410.

Norman, W. T. (1963). Toward an adequate taxonomy of personality attributes: Replicated factor structure in peer nomination personality ratings. *Journal of Abnormal and Social Psychology, 66,* 547–583.

Northouse, P. (2010). *Leadership: Theory and practice* (5th ed.). Thousand Oaks, CA: Sage.

Rowold, J., & Heinitz, K. (2007). Transformational and charismatic leadership: Assessing the convergent, divergent and criterion validity of the MLQ and the CKS. *Leadership Quarterly, 18,* 121–133.

Salovey, P., & Mayer, J. (1990). Emotional intelligence. *Imagination, Cognition, and Personality, 9,* 185–211.

Shamir, B., House, R. J., & Arthur, M. B. (1993). The motivational effects of charismatic leadership: A self-concept based theory. *Organization Science, 4*(4), 577–594.

Sparrowe, R. T., Soetjipto, B. W., & Kraimer, M. L. (2006). Do leaders' influence tactics relate to members' helping behavior? It depends on the quality of the relationship. *Academy of Management Journal, 49*(6), 1194–1208.

Stogdill, R. M. (1948). Personal factors associated with leadership: A survey of the literature. *Journal of Psychology, 25,* 35–71.

Stogdill, R. M. (1974). *Handbook of leadership: A survey of theory and research.* New York, NY: Free Press.

Van Rooy, D. L., & Viswesvaran, C. (2004). Emotional intelligence: A meta-analytic investigation of predictive validity and nomological net. *Journal of Vocational Behavior, 65,* 71–95.

Waldman, D. A., Javidan, M., & Varella, P. (2004). Charismatic leadership at the strategic level: A new application of upper echelons theory. *Leadership Quarterly, 15,* 355–380.

Weber, M. (1947). *The theory of social and economic organization* (T. Parson, Trans.). New York, NY: Free Press.

Wolff, S. B., Pescosolido, A. T., & Druskat, V. U. (2002). Emotional intelligence as the basis of leadership emergence in self-managing teams. *Leadership Quarterly, 13*, 505–522.

Wong, C. S., & Law, K. S. (2002). The effects of leader and follower emotional intelligence on performance and attitude: An exploratory study. *Leadership Quarterly, 13*, 243–274.

Yukl, G. (1999). An evaluation of conceptual weaknesses in transformational and charismatic leadership theories. *Leadership Quarterly, 10*, 285–305.

Yukl, G. (2010). *Leadership in organizations* (7th ed.). Upper Saddle River, NJ: Prentice Hall.

Yukl, G., Chavez, C., & Seifert, C. F. (2005). Assessing the construct validity and utility of two new influence tactics. *Journal of Organizational Behavior, 26*(6), 705–725.

Yukl, G., & Falbe, C. M. (1990). Influence tactics and objectives in upward, downward and lateral influence attempts. *Journal of Applied Psychology, 75*(2), 132–140.

Yukl, G., Falbe, C. M., & Youn, J. Y. (1993). Patterns of influence behavior for managers. *Group & Organization Management, 18*(1), 5–28.

Yukl, G., Kim, H., & Falbe, C. M. (1996). Antecedents of influence outcomes. *Journal of Applied Psychology, 81*, 309–317.

Yukl, G., Lepsinger, R., & Lucia, A. (1992). Preliminary report on development and validation of the influence behavior questionnaire. In K. Clark, M. B. Clark, & D. P. Campbell (Eds.), *Impact of leadership* (pp. 417–427). Greensboro, NC: Center for Creative Leadership.

Yukl, G., Seifert, C. F., & Chavez, C. (2008). Validation of the extended influence behavior questionnaire. *Leadership Quarterly, 19*, 609–621.

Yukl, G., & Tracey, J. B. (1990). Consequences of influence tactics used with subordinates, peers and the boss. *Journal of Applied Psychology, 77*(4), 525–535.

CHAPTER

5

Early Contingency Models and Theories of Leadership

Brent J. Goertzen

I think there are particular people that others will follow, for whatever reason. Perhaps they have a sense of humour, they like their style.

When you look at organising events it's somebody who's got what is termed as "leadership qualities," they are people who are willing to tell other people what to do but have the respect of other people as well, or gain that respect.

Michele Erina Doyle and Mark K. Smith
(from *http://www.infed.org/leadership/traditional_leadership.htm*)

INTRODUCTION

Contingency leadership theories were developed by scholars to provide insight into how a given situation can affect the leadership process. The primary aim of these theories was to offer an understanding of which leadership style is optimal in a given situation. Many contingency and other situational leadership perspectives emerged in the 1960s and 1970s but were still popular in the 1980s. Despite the valuable contributions of these models to the understanding of leadership theory and practice, contingency and situational perspectives have received less attention in recent decades as research has turned to other areas of leadership investigation.

These theories describe how different aspects of a situation can enhance or neutralize leaders' ability to influence employee performance or other organizational outcomes. This chapter describes five contingency theories of leadership: (1) least preferred coworker (LPC) contingency model, (2) path–goal theory, (3) situational leadership theory, (4) normative decision-making model, and (5) substitutes or neutralizers for leadership.

LPC CONTINGENCY MODEL

The LPC contingency model of leadership postulates that performance of interacting groups is contingent on the interaction between leadership style and situational favorableness (Fiedler, 1964, 1971). The contingency theory is based on the presumption that neither leader characteristics nor situational factors alone can predict leadership effectiveness (Ayman, Chemers, & Fiedler, 1995). Previous leadership theories focused exclusively on the one-to-one relationships between a leader and an employee. The contingency model broadened previous conceptualizations of leadership by examining the role of the leader in influencing interacting groups. According to Fiedler, interacting groups are defined as groups whose members worked interdependently and cooperatively on common tasks.

Drawing on prior leader behavior theories, the LPC contingency model asserts that leaders typically demonstrate one of two general categories of behavior: task oriented or relationship oriented. Task-oriented leaders are generally concerned with reaching stated goals and objectives. Relationship-oriented leaders typically focus on the quality of the interpersonal relationship.

An individual's predominant leadership style is predicted by the LPC survey instrument. The score for the survey is obtained by asking the individual to think of all the coworkers he or she has ever worked with and select the one with whom he or she has been least able to work. Individuals respond to bipolar adjectives (e.g., friendly–unfriendly) on an eight-point scale to calculate a score regarding the quality of the relationship with the LPC. The LPC reflects the attitude of the leader toward the individual he or she finds most difficult to work with (Fiedler, 1978).

The LPC score indicates a leader's motive hierarchy. Individuals who score high in LPC are considered relationship oriented; they give highest priority to close and emotionally supportive relationships with employees. Task accomplishment is a secondary motivation that becomes important only after the primary motivation of supportive interpersonal relationships is fulfilled. Leaders who score low in LPC are considered task-oriented leaders; their primary concern is task accomplishment. The secondary motivation of interpersonal relationships becomes important only when the group is performing well or when risks or other threats toward task accomplishment have been minimized.

Leadership Points to Ponder

The productivity and competitive problems American manufacturers face result from ineffective top management, petrified in place, unwilling to accept change, failing to provide vision and leadership.

Phillip Alspach, President, Intercom, Inc. (from *Harvard Business Review*, November/December 1986)

Situational Favorableness Variables

Situational favorableness is broadly defined as "the degree to which the situation itself provides the leader with potential power and influence over the group's behavior" (Fiedler, 1971, p. 129). The LPC contingency model is comprised of three critical situational variables: (1) leader–member relations, (2) task structure, and (3) position power. "Leader–member relations" refers to the quality of the relationship between leaders and their employees. Good relations are characterized by friendliness, cooperation, and loyalty. Leader–member relations is considered to be the most important of the three variables that affect situational favorableness. "Task structure" is the extent to which the goals are clearly defined and how detailed the procedures are for tasks. "Position power" is the extent to which the leader has formal authority to evaluate employee performance and administer rewards and punishments.

The combination of the three situational variables determines the level of situational favorableness (**FIGURE 5-1**). A total of eight combinations of situational favorableness range on a continuum from very favorable (octant 1) to very unfavorable (octant 8). For example, a situation is considered highly favorable (e.g., octant 1) when the quality of leader–member relationships is strong, the task structure is high, and the leader can exercise strong control over tasks and personnel. However, a very unfavorable situation occurs when leader–member relationships are poor, the task is unstructured, and the leader possesses limited authority over the group (e.g., octant 8).

The LPC contingency theory is known as a leader-match theory in that the model predicts the types of situations in which the two leadership styles will likely be

Leader–Member Relations	Good				Poor			
Task Structure	**Structured**		**Unstructured**		**Structured**		**Unstructured**	
Position Power	Strong	Weak	Strong	Weak	Strong	Weak	Strong	Weak
	Very Favorable				Very Unfavorable			
Octant	1	2	3	4	5	6	7	8
Effective Leader	Low LPC	Low LPC	Low LPC	Low LPC	High LPC	High LPC	High LPC	Low LPC

Source: Fiedler (1967).

Figure 5-1 Variables that determine the level of situational favorableness.

effective. Effectiveness for this leadership theory is defined in terms of group performance of assigned tasks. Fiedler (1971) indicated that low-LPC (task-oriented) leaders are more effective in very favorable and very unfavorable situations, compared to high-LPC (relationship-oriented) leaders. However, in situations with moderate favorableness, high-LPC leaders are more effective than low-LPC leaders. Furthermore, the model predicts that leader effectiveness decreases as the "leader moves into a zone of situational control that does not match his or her LPC score" (Fiedler & Garcia, 1987, p. 83).

Research on LPC Contingency Model

Research regarding the model's ability to predict leader effectiveness has produced generally favorable results. In 1981, Strube and Garcia conducted a review of all published studies of the LPC contingency model and found strong overall support for the model. All but octant 2 were consistent with the model's propositions. Several years later, another meta-analysis reviewed all published studies and found general overall support for the model across the octants (Peters, Hartke, & Pohlmann, 1985).

Another meta-analysis conducted a decade later found that only "high-LPC and low-LPC leaders appear to have octants (7 and 1, respectively) in which they are clearly more effective than other leaders" (Schriesheim, Tepper, & Tetrault, 1994, p. 570).

Strengths

The LPC contingency model of leadership possesses several notable strengths. It was one of the first models that challenged scholars and practitioners to consider the impact of the situation on leaders. For several decades the model was the focus of a substantial number of research studies that examined the role of situational favorableness on leadership effectiveness (e.g., Peters et al., 1985). As such, the contingency model challenged the understanding of leadership by predicting how situational aspects influence the relationship between leadership style and group effectiveness. Despite early interest by scholars and practitioners, research regarding the model has waned in the decades since.

The LPC contingency model is predictive and provides valuable information about the type of leadership that is likely to be most effective in a given situation

(Northouse, 2010). As such, evaluating the three aspects of the situation, one is able to know which type of leader behavior is likely to be more effective in promoting group performance.

Additionally, the model presumes that leaders do not need to be effective in all situations. Northouse (2010) noted that too often "leaders in organizations feel the need to be *all things to all people*" (emphasis added; p. 115). These are exceptionally high expectations. The contingency model asserts that leaders will not be (and by extension should not be expected to be) effective in all situations. Rather, organizations ought to match leaders to optimal situations to fit their predominate leadership style.

Weaknesses and Limitations

The contingency model of leadership has received much criticism in the research literature. First, it fails to adequately explain why some leader styles are successful in some situations over others. A second major criticism pertains to the LPC survey. It does not seem to be valid on the surface. The LPC bases a person's overarching leadership style on the quality of the working relationship with his or her least preferred coworker. Furthermore, the LPC model presumes that an individual's leadership style is a relatively unchanging variable.

Additionally, the model fails to explain how three aspects of situational favorableness combine into a single dimension along a continuum. Scholars have noted that the weights used to combine the variables to create the octants seem arbitrary (Shiflett, 1973).

Another important criticism is that the model fails to explain what organizations should do when there is a mismatch between a leader's style and the workplace situation. The LPC is largely a personality theory in that the LPC assesses a leader's motivation hierarchy; it does not allow much room for how leaders can adapt their style to the situation. Rather, proponents of the model suggest "situation engineering" to modify the situation to better fit a leader's predominate style (Fiedler & Chemers, 1982). For example, for some leaders it may be to their advantage to make the leader–member relations worse to better fit the situation. However, this seems unethical and unwise (Schriesheim & Kerr, 1977).

Finally, much of the research regarding the model neglects leaders with medium LPC scores (Yukl, 2010). Some research suggests that medium-LPC leaders were actually more effective than low- and high-LPC leaders on five of the eight octants. This is presumably because of their balanced concern for both the relationships and the tasks (Kennedy, 1982).

Interest in the contingency model of leadership has diminished substantially over the past several decades, perhaps because of the advent of better situational models. However, the contingency model was one of the first leadership models to incorporate situational variables. A major contribution of the contingency model was to stimulate further interest on the part of both scholars and practitioners in examining these and other situational factors to advance the understanding of leadership (Yukl, 2010).

PATH-GOAL THEORY

The path–goal theory of leadership was designed to explain how leaders motivate subordinates to accomplish task-specific outcomes. Path–goal theory is largely influenced by expectancy theory, suggesting that behavior is a function of a specific outcome and that the outcome is sufficiently desirable to influence the behavior (House, 1971). The perceived probability of the outcome is called "expectancy," and the desirability of the outcome is called "valence."

House (1971) asserted that "the motivational functions of the leader consist of increasing personal payoffs to subordinates for work-goal attainment, and making the path to these payoffs easier to travel by clarifying it, reducing road blocks and pitfalls, and increasing the opportunities for personal satisfaction en route" (p. 324). Essentially, the key assumption of path–goal leadership theory is that leaders' behavior enhances subordinate motivation if subordinates believe they can perform their work, if their successful accomplishment of the work will lead to desired outcomes, and if those outcomes are meaningful to the subordinates. The challenge for leaders is to make use of a leadership style that best meets the motivational needs of subordinates.

Leadership Points to Ponder

Good leaders make people feel that they're at the very heart of things, not at the periphery. Everyone feels that he or she makes a difference to the success of the organization. When that happens people feel centered and that gives their work meaning.

Warren G. Bennis (from *http://thinkexist.com*)

Leader Behaviors

The original path–goal theory of leader effectiveness asserted four general categories of leader behavior: (1) directive, (2) supportive, (3) participative, and (4) achievement oriented. "Directive behaviors" are related to the leader providing psychological structure for subordinates, such as letting them know what is expected of them, scheduling work, giving specific guidance, and clarifying policies and procedures (Yukl, 2010). "Supportive behaviors" are associated with satisfying subordinates' needs. These behaviors include demonstrating concern for their welfare and creating a friendly and caring work environment. "Participative behaviors" are intended to encourage subordinate opinion and influence in decision-making processes. "Achievement-oriented behaviors" relate to encouraging performance by setting challenging goals, emphasizing excellence, and demonstrating confidence in employees in the attainment of high standards.

Employee and Task Characteristics

Path–goal leadership theory also asserts the importance of employee and task characteristics. These variables directly affect how a leader influences employees' motivation.

Research regarding path–goal leadership theory has examined employee factors, such as need for affiliation, preferences for structure, desire for control, and self-perceived ability. For example, employees who possess a high need for affiliation likely prefer supportive leader behaviors because they demonstrate friendship and personal concern on the part of the leader. However, employees who are authoritarian but have to work in uncertain situations prefer directive leader behaviors because of the psychological structure provided by the leader. Employees with a high internal locus of control prefer a participative leadership style because it allows them to feel in charge of their work. However, employees with an external locus of control may respond more favorably to a directive leadership approach because such employees believe that external forces greatly affect their circumstances. Self-perceived ability can also affect leaders' ability to influence employee motivation. Typically, as employees' perception of their ability increases, the need for directive leadership decreases (Northouse, 2007).

Task characteristics can also influence leaders' ability to influence employee satisfaction and effort. Task characteristics include such aspects as task design (structure), formal authority, and primary work groups (**FIGURE 5-2**). In situations where the task is ambiguous and unstructured, directive leader behaviors may be necessary to provide employees with the needed clarity. Where group norms are weak and lack cohesion, supportive leader behaviors may provide needed encouragement.

Directive leader behaviors were proposed to have a positive effect on subordinate effort when tasks are ambiguous or when organizational policies or procedures are unclear (House & Mitchell, 1974). Additionally, directive leader behaviors can increase the size of the incentive or strengthen reward contingencies (Yukl, 2010).

Supportive leader behaviors were postulated to be most effective in promoting satisfaction for subordinates who work in stressful or frustrating tasks (House & Mitchell, 1974). The supportive behaviors help reduce the level of subordinate anxiety and minimize the unpleasant aspects of the work and enhance employees' self-confidence (Yukl, 2010). However, if employees are already interested in aspects of the job or have a high level of self-confidence, the supportive leader behavior likely has a negligible effect on their satisfaction or performance.

Participative leader behaviors provide subordinates with opportunities to become involved in the decision-making processes that directly affect their work. It has been postulated that participative leader behaviors enhance subordinate effort and satisfaction when tasks are unstructured. This process helps subordinates clarify roles and responsibilities. However, when tasks are highly structured, participative behaviors are thought to have little effect. Participative behaviors may also increase valence among employees who possess a high need for achievement and autonomy (Yukl, 2010).

Achievement-oriented behaviors are intended to help followers set challenging goals and communicate the expectation that followers perform at their highest levels. House & Mitchell (1974) proposed that these behaviors would increase employee satisfaction and effort when tasks are ambiguous and nonrepetitive. However, it was expected that achievement-oriented behaviors would not increase employee effort or satisfaction for tasks that were structured or repetitive.

Research on the Theory

Research regarding the path–goal theory of leadership has produced mixed results. Wofford and Liska (1993) conducted a meta-analysis of 120 studies and Podsakoff, MacKenzie, Ahearne, and Bommer (1995) extensively reviewed the research. Despite the large number of studies, many of the results were inconclusive because only a few of the propositions between leader behavior and employee performance and satisfaction were statistically significant.

Strengths

Path–goal theory is the first leadership theory to specify four categories of leader behavior (directive, supportive, participative, and achievement oriented) that offer more specific and refined definitions. All previous research focused on two primary categories of leader behavior: task- and relationship-oriented behaviors (Jermier,

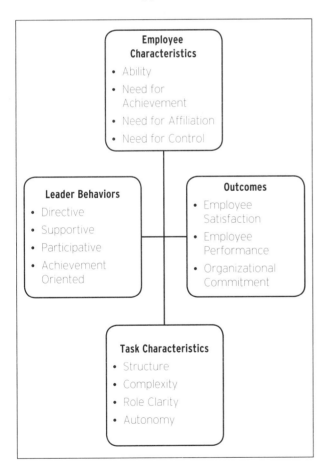

Figure 5-2 Path-goal leadership theory.

1996). Additionally, path–goal theory of leadership is one of the first situational contingency theories to explore the impact of employee characteristics and task characteristics on leaders' ability to influence employee satisfaction and performance.

The path–goal theory focuses on the motivation principles of expectancy theory. According to Northouse (2010), no other leadership theory directly deals with follower motivation in this way. As such, the theory requires leaders to continually ask themselves questions about how to improve the payoffs for employees; how to "clear the path" for them to accomplish their work; how to help them feel they have the confidence to do the work; how to ensure that if they do the work they will be rewarded with meaningful incentives.

Path–goal theory presumes that leaders can, and must, adapt their behaviors based on the style that best fits the needs and characteristics of employees and the given task characteristics. Thus, this leadership theory is pragmatic in that it emphasizes various ways by which leaders can increase followers' motivation by identifying meaningful rewards and helping them achieve goals.

Weaknesses and Limitations

There are several limitations to the path–goal leadership theory, most notably the lack of empirical research to support the theory's propositions. Despite the many studies that have been conducted, there has been limited support in the research for the model. Some studies have found a relationship between leader directiveness and employee satisfaction; however, other studies have not confirmed the relationship. Additionally, some leadership styles have received more attention than others. For instance, comparatively more studies have examined leader directive and supportive behaviors, whereas not enough studies have adequately examined participative and achievement-oriented leader behaviors (Podsakoff et al., 1995).

Although the theory is pragmatic, it is also complex. Knowing how to simultaneously integrate employee characteristics in concert with various task characteristics to determine appropriate leadership style to match the situation is a daunting task. The theory is comprised of a broad set of assumptions and propositions, which makes it extremely difficult to use the theory to improve leadership processes in organizations (Northouse, 2010).

Additionally, path–goal theory has been criticized on grounds of conceptual weaknesses. Path–goal relies heavily on broad categories of leader behavior. Examining more specific behaviors, such as "clarifying role expectations," "recognizing accomplishments," and "communicating high expectations," may provide more clear links between leader influence attempts and employee motivation (Yukl, 2010).

Another criticism of path–goal theory is that it treats leadership as a one-way event (Northouse, 2007). The theory describes the importance of leaders' role in providing guidance, direction, and support to employees and helping them remove obstacles as they reach their goals. This theory has the potential to create dependency on leaders because essentially all of the responsibility is on them. Employees' only role to the organization and contribution to the leadership process is that of achieving performance outcomes.

SITUATIONAL LEADERSHIP MODEL

Situational leadership is one of the first models to examine leadership beyond simply the qualities (e.g., traits) of leaders or their behaviors. Scholars acknowledge the relevance of various situational aspects (e.g., leaders, followers, organization, job demands, and time) that can influence the leadership process. Originators of the situational leadership theory focused primarily on developing a predictive model of the influence of leader behavior on follower readiness.

Readiness is defined as "the extent to which a follower has the ability and willingness to accomplish a specific task" (Hersey & Blanchard, 1993, p. 189). Readiness can be viewed as either an individual or group-level phenomenon, depending on the nature of the tasks being accomplished and the interdependent functioning of the group. Still, although the group as a whole may be at one readiness level, individuals within that group may be at another.

Readiness comprises two components: job readiness (ability) and psychological readiness (willingness). Job readiness involves possessing the knowledge and skills necessary to complete a given task. Individuals with a high level of job readiness in a given area have the ability to complete objectives without guidance from others. Psychological readiness relates to the willingness and motivation of the follower to do something. Psychological readiness involves both confidence and commitment. Individuals with high levels of psychological readiness possess high self-confidence regarding that particular aspect of their jobs and do not need excessive encouragement to accomplish things in that area.

The two dimensions of follower readiness yield four possible readiness levels: (1) Low readiness (R1) describes an employee who is both unable and unwilling to accomplish the task in the given area. (2) Low to moderate readiness (R2) is characterized as the employee being unable but willing to perform the given assignment. (3) Moderate to high readiness (R3) is represented by an employee who possesses high job readiness (ability) yet is insecure or unwilling to perform the task. (4) High readiness (R4) corresponds to an employee who demonstrates both the ability and willingness to accomplish the given job responsibility (**TABLE 5-1**).

The situational leadership model draws on previous research (Stogdill & Coons, 1957) regarding both task-oriented and relationship-oriented leader behaviors. The model presumes that task-oriented and relationship-oriented behaviors are two independent dimensions. The task-oriented approach includes specific behaviors, such as goal setting, organizing, setting time lines, directing, and controlling. The relationship-oriented style involves such activities as giving support, communicating, facilitating interaction, active listening, and providing feedback (Hersey & Blanchard, 1982). Combining high–low levels of the behavior type along each dimension yields four categories of leader style: (1) telling, (2) selling, (3) participating, and (4) delegating (**FIGURE 5-3**).

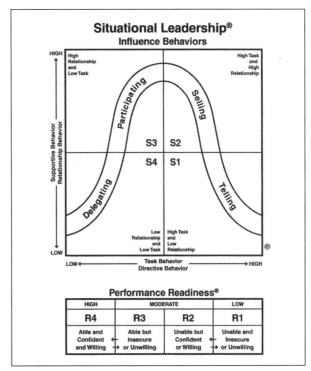

Figure 5-3 Situational leadership model.

Telling (S1) is characterized by high task-oriented and low relationship-oriented behavior and is described as providing clear, specific directions. It emphasizes directive behavior that clearly defines followers' roles and the "what" and "how" of various tasks. This style best fits the employee who lacks both the confidence and ability (low readiness) to perform a given task.

Table 5-1 Leader Behavior Appropriate for Various Readiness Levels

Readiness Level	Appropriate Leader Behavior
R1: Low readiness Unable and unwilling or insecure	S1: Telling High task and low relationship behavior
R2: Low to moderate readiness Unable but willing or confident	S2: Selling High task and high relationship behavior
R3: Moderate to high readiness Able but unwilling to insecure	S3: Participating High relationship and low task behavior
R4: High readiness Able/competent and willing/confident	S4: Delegating Low relationship and low task behavior

Source: Hersey and Blanchard, 1993.

Selling (S2) behavior combines high task and relationship behaviors. This approach is best suited for followers who possess confidence in themselves yet lack the necessary knowledge or skills to achieve the objective. The supportive behavior reinforces followers' confidence, and the directive behavior provides them with the necessary ability to get the job done.

Participating (S3) describes a blend of high relationship-oriented and low task-oriented behaviors. This supportive and nondirective style best fits followers who demonstrate moderate to high readiness in that they are able to perform the given assignment (job readiness), but simply lack the self-confidence (psychological readiness) to achieve the goal. This classification of leader behavior is "participating" because, although the main role of the leader is to facilitate the communication process, the leader and followers should share in decision making.

Delegating (S4) combines limited task-oriented and relationship-oriented behaviors. Because high-readiness followers possess both ability and willingness, little guidance and support are necessary to achieve the desired outcome. The leader may still provide followers with the problem, but highly mature followers provide the necessary "how" and "where" to complete the task.

Application of the Model

The situational leadership perspective presumes that followers move backward and forward along the readiness continuum depending on their level of comfort and ability with given tasks. For leaders to be effective, they must be able to accurately assess follower readiness and apply appropriate leadership styles to meet their needs.

The first step in applying the model is to determine the readiness level of followers by making a judgment about their levels of ability and motivation. Information about readiness levels can be gained by asking people directly and by observing behavior. One could ask such questions as, "How well do you think you are doing this?" or "How enthusiastic are you about . . . ?" Or leaders may determine both willingness and ability by observing past performance in areas that might relate to the given task. Regardless of the technique used to assess follower readiness level, leaders must be able to evaluate the following issues: Does the follower possess sufficient skills and willingness to accomplish the tasks?

The next step is to adapt the leadership style to match follower readiness. For instance, new employees who may lack security in their abilities and may lack the knowledge to complete an assignment (R1) need minimal supportive but high directive assistance from their supervisor (S1: telling). However, seasoned organizational members who have demonstrated both the desire and competence to fulfill their responsibilities in a given area (R4) need minimal guidance and limited support (S4: delegating) from their supervisors.

It is important for leaders to understand that followers can move backward and forward along the readiness continuum as job assignments change. Therefore, it is critical that leaders be flexible in adapting their leadership styles to suit the readiness levels of individuals or their work group. Not all individuals progress through the readiness levels at the same pace. Some may move rather quickly to higher levels of readiness and others more slowly. Readiness levels may decrease, especially if organizations change modes of operation that require employees to adapt to new job responsibilities or ways of organizing work.

Leaders play an important role in developing the readiness level of followers (Hersey & Blanchard, 1993). Leaders do this by providing more and more responsibility to the individual or group and providing appropriate leadership styles until the level of performance expectations are met.

Strengths

Situational leadership is a widely used and popular leadership model, especially for leadership practitioners (Northouse, 2007). It served as the basis for many training and development programs to develop leaders within organizations. Perhaps it has gained wide credibility and acceptance among practitioners because of its intuitive approach to leadership. The situational leadership model is a relatively simple approach compared to other leadership models (e.g., LPC contingency model in Fiedler, 1971). Furthermore, it is relatively easy to apply across settings, such as work and family.

It presumes that leaders can and must adapt their styles to employees at different readiness levels (Graeff, 1983). Leaders must be flexible and not rely solely on one predominant leadership approach to all individuals across all situations. Effective leaders make appropriate use of each leadership style according to the situation.

As such, another strength of the situational leadership theory is its prescriptive ability (Northouse, 2007). It provides clear direction on which leadership style is effective for task requirements based on employees' needs. Furthermore, the model requires leaders to treat employees differently, based on their readiness levels, and provide them with opportunities to develop their abilities and confidence in their work (Fernandez & Vecchio, 1997).

Weaknesses and Limitations

The situational approach is not without its limitations. Perhaps most notably, although practitioners have widely accepted the model as a credible leadership theory, few empirical studies have investigated this approach. The lack of a strong body of research raises questions about the theory's assumptions and tenets. Many of the studies testing the propositions of the model are unpublished dissertations; the few published studies "at best, provide limited support for the validity" of the situational leadership theory (Graeff, 1997). For example, Vecchio (1987) conducted a study of more than 300 high school teachers and their principals. The study concluded that teachers were more satisfied and performed better with principals who use a more directive leadership style. However, performance was unrelated to principal style among more mature and experienced teachers. In general, there is a lack of empirical support for few of the situational leadership propositions (Blank, Weitzel, & Green 1990; Thompson & Vecchio, 2009).

Another limitation of situational leadership is the ambiguity of several critical concepts. For example, psychological readiness and job readiness are treated together as a global concept of readiness. Psychological readiness is asserted as a continuum from unwilling to willing (Hersey & Blanchard, 1982). However, there is an internal consistency problem because the R3 level of readiness asserts that employees may be less willing than individuals at the R2 level (Graeff, 1997).

Other versions of the situational leadership model (SLII: Blanchard, 1985) changed the readiness levels to developmental levels: D1, low competence and high commitment; D2, low competence and low commitment; D3, moderate to high competence and low commitment; and D4, high competence and high commitment. The SLII also labeled the classifications of leadership styles slightly differently but still retained the general tenets of task-oriented and relationship-oriented behaviors. However, the authors do not make it clear how or why competence combines with commitment into these categories (Northouse, 2007).

Furthermore, the situational leadership model fails to account for important demographic factors (e.g., age or gender) that influence the leader–follower prescriptions. Vecchio and Boatwright (2002) found that age was positively related to structure; older employees tend to desire more structure than younger employees. Additionally, female employees preferred more supportive behaviors and male employees tended to prefer a more directive leadership style.

Another limitation of the situational leadership model is that it views leadership as a unidirectional influence process, as something that leaders do to followers to accomplish tasks through their efforts.

NORMATIVE DECISION-MAKING MODEL

Decision making has been recognized as a critical component of leadership processes for many years. Vroom and Yetton (1973) developed a rational decision-making model that increases the likeliness of decision effectiveness for a given situation. This model attempts to prescribe decision-making methods most appropriate for a given situation. The model asserts two classes of outcomes that affect decision effectiveness: the quality or rationality of the decision, and acceptance or commitment by employees to execute the decision.

Decision Quality

Decision quality depends on where relevant information for a given problem resides. Does the leader have all of the relevant information to make the decision? Can employees provide not only pertinent, but also critical, information that can influence the quality of the decision? The model presumes that employees who possess relevant information are willing to cooperate in the decision-making and implementation processes (Yukl, 2010). When leaders and employees share in the organization's objectives, consultation and group decision processes equally facilitate decision quality.

However, when employees' goals are not compatible with the goals of the leader or organization, then group decision making is eliminated from the feasible set of decision style options.

Acceptance

Decision acceptance refers to the level of commitment needed to implement a decision effectively. The model generally presumes that greater employee participation in the decision process increases the acceptance of the decision. If acceptance is not a priority, then autocratic decision style is preferred. However, if the implementation of the decision requires employee buy-in or in other ways may affect employee motivation, then leaders should use decision styles that require their involvement. Also, if acceptance is necessary and there are substantial differences in opinions of employees, participation can help resolve the disagreements with full knowledge of the problem.

There are five categories of decision procedures, each with varying levels of involvement and participation of employees: two varieties of autocratic; two varieties of consultative; and one type of joint decision making (group) between leaders and followers. **TABLE 5-2** defines each of the decision processes (A stands for autocratic, C for consultative, and G for group).

The model integrates situational variables, which are often framed in a series of eight yes/no diagnostic questions. The diagnostic questions are identified in **TABLE 5-3**. Answers to these questions determine the problem type, which then yields a set of decision styles (called a feasibility set) that likely leads to successful solutions. The feasibility set is defined as "the methods that remain after all those which violate rules designated to protect the quality and acceptance of the decision have been excluded" (Vroom & Yetton, 1973, p. 37).

Decision Rules

The Vroom–Yetton model (**FIGURE 5-4**) provides a set of rules intended to protect both the quality and acceptance of the decision by eliminating inappropriate decision styles for a given situation. The rules are summarized briefly in **TABLE 5-4**. For several problem types, there are several decision procedures in the feasibility set (**TABLE 5-5**). In those situations, decision procedure criteria should be based on other factors, such as time pressure or personal preference of the leader.

In general, autocratic decision-making style is appropriate when:

1. The leader has sufficient information
2. The quality of the decision is not essential
3. Employees do not agree with one another

Table 5-2 Types of Leadership Decision Styles

AI	You solve the problem or make the decision yourself, using information available to you at that time.
AII	You obtain necessary information from your employee(s) and then decide on the solution to the problem yourself. You may or may not tell your employees what the problem is in getting the information from them. The role played by your employees is clearly one of providing the necessary information to you, rather than generating or evaluating alternative solutions.
CI	You share the problem with relevant employees individually, getting their ideas and suggestions without bringing them together as a group. Then you make the decision that may or may not reflect your employees' influence.
CII	You share the problem with your employees as a group, collectively obtaining their ideas and suggestions. Then you make the decision that may or may not reflect your employees' influence.
GII	You share the problem with your employees as a group. Together you generate and evaluate alternatives and attempt to reach agreement (consensus) on a solution. Your role is much like that of chairman. You do not try to influence the group to adopt a particular solution, and you are willing to accept and implement any solution that has the support of the entire group.

Source: Table 2.1. "Decision Methods for Group and Individual Problems," from *Leadership and Decision-Making*, by Victor H. Vroom and Philip W. Yetton, © 1973. Reprinted by permission of the University of Pittsburgh Press.

Table 5-3 Diagnostic Questions

A	If the decision were accepted, would it make a difference which course of action were adopted?
B	Do I have sufficient information to make a high-quality decision?
C	Do employees have sufficient additional information to result in high-quality decision?
D	Do I know exactly what information is needed, who possesses it, and how to collect it?
E	Is acceptance of decision by subordinates critical to effective implementation?
F	If I were to make the decision myself, is it certain that it would be accepted by my employees?
G	Can employees be trusted to base solutions on organizational considerations?
H	Is conflict among employees likely in preferred solutions?

Source: Table 2.3. "Problem Attributes," from *Leadership and Decision-Making*, by Victor H. Vroom and Philip W. Yetton, © 1973. Reprinted by permission of the University of Pittsburgh Press.

4. Employees do not agree with the goals of the organization

Consultative decision styles are better suited in situations when:

1. The leader has sufficient information, but employees strongly desire participation

2. The leader has insufficient information and consultation will provide the leader with the necessary information

3. Employees generally agree with organizational goals

Group-oriented decision styles are better suited in situations when:

1. The leader does not have all relevant information

2. Quality is important

3. Employee commitment is important

There are several practical implications of the model for managers in organizations. First, managers must be able to understand the situation and determine when to

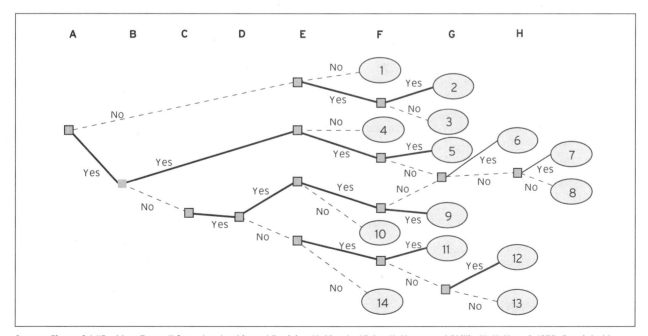

Source: Figure 3.1 "Problem Types," from *Leadership and Decision-Making*, by Victor H. Vroom and Phillip W. Yetton, © 1973. Reprinted by permission of the University of Pittsburgh Press.

Figure 5-4 Decision tree of the Vroom and Yetton model.

Table 5-4 Decision Rules

Rules to Protect Quality
Leader Information Rule: If quality of decision is important and leader does not possess enough information/ expertise, then AI is eliminated from feasibility set.
Goal Congruence Rule: If quality of decision is important and employees are not likely to pursue organizational goals, then GII is eliminated from feasibility set.
Unstructured Rule: If quality is important, if leader lacks necessary information, and if problem is unstructured and employees possess relevant information, then AI, AII, and CI are eliminated from feasibility set.
Rules to Protect Acceptance
Acceptance Rule: If acceptance is critical and it's not certain that an autocratic decision will be accepted, then AI and AII are eliminated from feasibility set.
Conflict Rule: If acceptance is critical, it's not certain that an autocratic decision will accepted, disagreements are likely, and decision methods would enable a resolution of differences with full knowledge of the problem, then AI, AII, and CI are eliminated from feasibility set.
Fairness Rule: If quality is unimportant but acceptance is critical, it's not certain that an autocratic decision will be accepted, and the decision requires employees to determine a fair method of resolving differences, then AI, AII, CI, and CII are eliminated from feasibility set.
Acceptance Priority Rule: If acceptance is critical, it's not certain that an autocratic decision will be accepted, certain employees will pursue organizational goals, and the decision process will provide acceptance without damaging quality, then AI, AII, CI, and CII are eliminated from feasibility set.

Source: Vroom & Jago, 1978, p. 153.

make use of different decision-making styles. Second, managers must realize that the group (participative) approach is not always best. Although participation may seem to be desirable, time constraints, potential conflict, and mismatch of organizational goals may impede decision quality.

Leadership Points to Ponder

The single biggest way to impact an organization is to focus on leadership development. There is almost no limit to the potential of an organization that recruits good people, raises them up as leaders, and continually develops them.

John C Maxwell: *The 17 Irrefutable Laws of Teamwork* (2001, p. 185)

Research on the Model

Much of the research regarding the Vroom–Yetton model involved field research whereby managers were asked to recall effective and ineffective decisions they had made and describe the situational aspects that contributed to the success (or lack thereof) of the implemented solution (Jago & Vroom, 1980; Tjosvold, Wedley, & Field, 1986; Vroom & Jago, 1978). The original studies found that decision-making behavior fell within the prescribed feasibility set 69% of the time (Vroom & Yetton, 1973). Field (1979) asserted that decision styles outside the feasibility set do not guarantee failure. Likewise, decisions made using approaches within the feasibility set do not guarantee success; however, they offer a higher probability of quality and acceptance.

One study indicated that although the Vroom–Yetton decision rules were supported, an alternative model was a better predictor of decision effectiveness. A decision-making process called "constructive controversy," whereby managers intentionally involve numerous personnel in discussions that involve opposing ideas and issues, was more predictive of successful decisions than the Vroom–Yetton model (Tjosvold et al., 1986). The authors of the study challenged the assumption that social interaction impedes decision making and asserted

Table 5-5 Problem Types and the Feasible Set of Decision Processes

Problem Type	Acceptable Methods
1	AI, AII, CI, CII, GII
2	AI, AII, CI, CII, GII
3	GII
4	AI, AII, CI, CII, GII*
5	AI, AII, CI, CII, GII*
6	GII
7	CII
8	CI, CII
9	AII, CI, CII, GII*
10	AII, CI, CII, GII*
11	CII, GII*
12	GII
13	CII
14	CII, GII*

*Within the feasible set only when the answer to question regarding compatibility of goals is "yes."

Source: Table 3.1. "Problem Types and Feasible Sets of Decision Methods," from *Leadership and Decision-Making*, by Victor H. Vroom and Philip W. Yetton, © 1973. Reprinted by permission of the University of Pittsburgh Press.

that constructive controversy can surpass the negative impact of face-to-face interactions.

Research indicated that leaders vary in the overall level of participation they use in decision making. However, the situation is often more important than level of decision in determining decision success (Vroom & Jago, 1988; Vroom & Jago, 2007; Vroom & Yetton, 1973). Furthermore, leaders often respond with combinations of situational dimensions (Jago, 1978). For instance, in situations when acceptance of decisions is important, leaders are often less participative if the issue is likely to cause conflict compared to situations when conflict is not expected. Leaders choose not to be participative, believing that the conflict may exacerbate the situation (Vroom & Jago, 2007). However, in situations where acceptance of decisions is immaterial, leaders often use a participative style for issues that may cause conflict, believing that the conflict could be constructive and otherwise enhance the quality of the decision without endangering acceptance of the decision.

The Vroom–Yetton decision-making model is imperfect. Overall, research has found some support for the model, but more research is required to sufficiently test all of the decision rules.

Weaknesses and Limitations

Several scholars have been critical of the normative decision-making model because of a number of conceptual weaknesses. For instance, decision processes in this model are viewed as discrete events that occur at a single point in time. However, many important decisions are not made this way (Yukl, 2010). Major decisions often require numerous meetings and involve various participants at different times throughout the decision cycle. As a result, a leader must make use of a series of different decision procedures with different people at different times throughout the decision cycle.

Field (1979) offered a critique of the Vroom–Yetton model and asserted that the model simply is not conceptually clear. There is distinction between the autocratic, consultative, and group decision processes. However, Field argued that the model fails to make clear distinctions between the subvarieties of each procedure (i.e., AI versus AII and CI versus CII). Furthermore, the original Vroom–Yetton model asserted that time was not a factor in the rules that govern effective decision making. Field reported that time is quite commonly an important resource expenditure. Additionally, the model asserts that employees may not act in accordance with the organization's goals but rather out of self-interest. The model does not account for a leader who may also act out of self-interest and therefore interfere with effective decisions.

Finally, the model presumes that leaders possess the necessary skills to effectively facilitate each type of decision-making process. Although the model held for skilled leaders, for unskilled leaders the model was exceedingly difficult to apply (Crouch & Yetton, 1987). Crouch and Yetton reported that unskilled leaders experienced a high performance cost, especially when situations involved conflict among employees that required high levels of consultative (CII) and joint decision making (GII).

THE SUBSTITUTES FOR LEADERSHIP MODEL

Kerr and Jermier (1978) developed a model of leadership that sought to explain how aspects of the situation can negate or even substitute for leadership. Their studies indicated that a wide variety of individual, task, and organizational characteristics influence the relationship between leader behaviors and employee satisfaction and performance. The model distinguishes between two types of situational variables: substitutes and neutralizers (TABLE 5-6). Neutralizers are characteristics that make it impossible for relationship- or task-oriented leadership to make an impact on employee performance and satisfaction. Substitutes are characteristics that "render

relationship- and/or task-oriented leadership not only impossible but also unnecessary" (p. 395).

> ## Leadership Points to Ponder
>
> *When the leadership is right and the time is right, the people can always be counted upon to follow—to the end and at all costs.*
>
> Harold J. Seymour
> (from *http://www.worldofquotes.com*)

Employee Characteristics

Certain characteristics of employees influence the ability of the leader to meaningfully affect employee performance and satisfaction. For example, employees who bring extensive training and experience do not require substantial supervision because they already possess the knowledge and skills necessary for the given job. Professional orientation refers to the desire to cultivate

Table 5-6 Substitutes and Neutralizers for Relationship and Task-Oriented Leadership

Substitute or Neutralizer	Relationship-Oriented Leadership	Task-Oriented Leadership
Employee Characteristics		
Experience, ability, training		Substitute
Professional orientation	Substitute	Substitute
Indifference toward rewards	Neutralizer	Neutralizer
Task Characteristics		
Structured, routine task		Substitute
Feedback provided by task		Substitute
Intrinsically satisfying task	Substitute	
Organization Characteristics		
Cohesive work group	Substitute	Substitute
Low position power	Neutralizer	Neutralizer
Formalization (roles, procedures)		Substitute
Inflexibility (rules, policies)		Neutralizer
Dispersed employee work sites	Neutralizer	Neutralizer

Source: Yukl, G. A., *Leadership in Organizations*, 7th Edition, © 2010, p. 237. Reprinted by permission of Pearson Education, Inc., Upper Saddle River, NJ.

"horizontal relationships" that give greater credence to peer review feedback, and developing relationships outside the organization through profession or industry associations and other such entities. These behaviors and attitudes reduce the need for hierarchical influence. Yukl (2010) reported that professionals, such as medical doctors, accountants, and airline pilots, do not require and often do not want much supervision.

Indifference toward rewards refers to the lack of enthusiasm toward rewards or opportunities provided by the organization. For instance, leaders should not attempt to provide employees with recognition and praise when they more highly value time off from work to be with their families.

Task Characteristics

Various aspects of the task can substitute for leader behavior. Simple and routine tasks essentially serve as a substitute for task-oriented guidance from the leader. These repetitive routines can easily be learned without extensive training from supervisors. Additionally, task-provided feedback is often the most immediate and accurate form of feedback and essentially reduces, if not eliminates, the need for leader-provided feedback for task-related performance issues. Also, the level of intrinsic satisfaction provided by employee tasks serves as a substitute for relationship-oriented behaviors; employees do not require inspiration and motivation from leaders because the tasks are intrinsically motivating.

Organization Characteristics

Among the organization characteristics that influence the relationship between leader behaviors and employee performance is the cohesiveness of the work group. The cooperative relationships among work group members likely provide the needed support from others and the task-relevant guidance necessary to effectively accomplish the performance objectives. Low position power refers to leaders' relatively limited ability to provide motivating rewards. Low position power neutralizes leaders' ability to influence employee performance and satisfaction.

Formalized roles and procedures often provide needed structure for job assignments and therefore substitute for leader task-oriented behavior. Inflexible rules can serve as both a substitute and neutralizer of leader

behaviors because there is limited room to make any task changes by the leader to help facilitate employee effort. Additionally, geographic dispersion of the employees and work sites affects the relationship between leader behavior and employee effort. Leader behaviors are neutralized in organizations where employees are geographically dispersed because there is infrequent contact with leaders.

Implications for Substitutes for Leadership Model

There are interesting implications of the substitutes for leadership model. Howell, Bowen, Dorfman, Kerr, and Podsakoff (1990) asserted that the primary advantage of the substitutes construct is that it identifies potential "remedies for problems stemming from weak leadership" (p. 24). Kerr and Jermier (1978) described the importance for organizations of providing both guidance and support to employees to maximize individual and organizational performance. However, prior leadership models presumed that those task-oriented and relationship-oriented behaviors would be provided almost exclusively by employees' supervisors. It is not necessary for supervisors to be the sole providers of guidance and support, but rather that these elements be provided somehow by the organization.

Supervisors (identified as "leader" by this model) do play a dominant role because there are frequent opportunities for downward influence in formal hierarchical relationships. Kerr and Jermier (1978) asserted that "few organizations would be expected to have leadership substitutes so strong as to totally overwhelm the leader, or so weak as to require subordinates to rely entirely on [the leader]. In most organizations it is likely that . . . substitutes exist for some leader activities but not for others" (p. 400).

How do leaders and organizations make use of the substitutes for leadership model? One approach is to train leaders to effectively evaluate situational aspects that have the potential to negate their influence attempts on employees. However, despite Kerr and Jermier's (1978) assertion, Howell and coworkers (1990) contend that some organizations may have so many neutralizers that it is nearly impossible for leaders to succeed. Therefore, another approach is to modify the neutralizers and create a more favorable situation in which the leader can succeed, such as increasing employees' perceptions of the leader's influence and expertise, building organizational climate, increasing employees' dependence on the leader, increasing the leader's position power, or creating cohesive work groups with high performance norms.

Additionally, organizations could make leadership less important by focusing more attention on substitutes (Yukl, 2010). Howell and coworkers (1990) describe several suggestions for an organization to create substitutes for leader task-oriented and relationship-oriented behaviors: develop collegial systems of guidance, improve a performance-oriented organizational culture, increase availability of administrative staff, increase professionalism of employees, redesign jobs, and start team-building activities to develop self-management skills.

Research on Leadership Substitutes

Numerous studies have been conducted regarding aspects of the substitutes for leadership model. "Despite widespread intuitive appeal, empirical support for the substitutes models has not been encouraging" (Podsakoff, MacKenzie, & Bommer, 1996, p. 380).

Podsakoff et al. (1996) conducted a comprehensive review of published studies regarding leadership substitutes. Their results indicate that substitutes generally do explain some of the variation between leader behaviors and employee satisfaction and performance. However, they concluded that substitutes do not serve as true moderators of the relationship between these variables as proposed in the theory. Furthermore, no studies have found a consistent pattern of these relationships.

More recently, scholars are calling for conceptual refinement and methodological improvement in the study of the substitutes for leadership model, because research supporting the model remains elusive (Dionne, Yammarino, Howell, & Villa, 2005). However, despite the lack of support for the theoretical model, there are sufficient data to indicate that substitutes for leadership are related to leader behavior and employee outcomes and that they should not be ignored as leadership variables (Podsakoff & MacKenzie, 1997).

Weaknesses and Limitations

The substitutes for leadership theory suffers from several important weaknesses. First, the model lacks a detailed rationale for the causal process for each of the proposed substitutes and neutralizers (Yukl, 2010). The ambiguity

has challenged researchers in developing testable propositions. Part of this ambiguity stems from a failure to differentiate direct actions by leaders on outcome variables (e.g., employee satisfaction and performance) from leaders' actions that influence situational characteristics, such as creating a cohesive environment or providing coaching by experienced team members to those with minimal experience.

Additionally, the model's theoretical basis requires refinement (Podsakoff, MacKenzie, & Fetter, 1993). A more clearly defined theory with added specificity could account for the direct and interactive effects of leader behavior and substitute aspects on organizational outcomes. Yukl (2010) asserted that broad, general categories of leader behavior, such as relationship-oriented and task-oriented behaviors, are limiting. More specific classifications of leader behavior (e.g., role clarifying or performance monitoring) will likely add the clarity needed to test the proposed moderating effects in the substitutes model.

Finally, many of the studies used survey instruments with poor psychometric properties (Williams et al., 1988). Attempts to refine such surveys have not been any more effective at detecting the moderating effects of the substitute constructs (e.g., Podsakoff et al., 1993). This may help explain the general lack of support for the model found in many studies. However, the lack of support may also be caused by other larger conceptual weakness.

SUMMARY

The earliest contingency theory of leadership is based on the work of Fiedler and colleagues, who developed the contingency model. They postulated that three critical aspects of the situation (leader–member relations, task structure, and position power) dictate which leadership style is effective. Task-oriented leaders are likely effective in highly favorable and unfavorable situations. Relationship-oriented leaders are likely effective only in moderately unfavorable situations.

Path–goal leadership theory emphasizes the importance of follower motivation and described how leaders can provide meaningful rewards to influence follower performance. Path–goal theory describes four categories of leader behavior: directive, supportive, participative, and achievement oriented. Effective leaders, according to this perspective, adopt the leadership style that is appropriate for their employees and task characteristics.

The situational leadership model, developed by Hersey and Blanchard, views the leadership context in terms of follower readiness. They believe that leaders must first understand an employee's level of confidence and ability to perform a given task, and then provide the appropriate level of guidance and encouragement that enables the employee to perform the task effectively.

Vroom and colleagues perceive leadership as based largely on decision-making processes. The normative decision-making model rests primarily on decision quality and acceptance and proposes a series of decision rules aimed at protecting these two critical facets of decision making. Based on the combination of decision rules, leaders are to use one of five categories of decision procedures, each with varying levels of employee involvement and participation: two varieties of autocratic; two varieties of consultative; and one type of joint decision making (group) between leaders and followers.

Developed by Kerr and Jermier, the substitutes and neutralizers theory of leadership explains how a variety of individual, task, and organizational characteristics affects how leaders promote organizational effectiveness. Neutralizers make it impossible for the leader to have an impact, whereas substitutes not only make it impossible for the leader to influence employees' performance, but also make their efforts unnecessary.

Wrap-Up

ACTIVITY

Situational Leadership

Part One:

The situational leadership model is based on the assumption that the leader's style must adapt to the readiness level of the follower. Identify and briefly describe a scenario for each of the four readiness levels described in the Hersey and Blanchard model.

Part Two:

This activity focuses on the application of the situational leadership model. First, consider your default leadership style. Which style do you use most commonly when attempting to influence employees to complete an assigned task? This style presumes a particular readiness level of the employee; describe the readiness level assumed with that style. Next, think of a particular time when you were successful in using that default style. How should your approach have been different if the employee possessed lower psychological readiness and job readiness? How should you have changed your approach if the employee held high psychological readiness and job readiness?

Substitutes and Neutralizers of Leadership

There are a variety of characteristics that can affect one's ability to engage in leadership in the workplace. Identified next are the aspects of situations that can either substitute for or neutralize the ability to engage in leadership in the workplace.

Employee characteristics
- Experience, ability, and training
- Professional orientation
- Attitude toward rewards

Task characteristics
- Structured, routine task
- Feedback provided by task
- Intrinsically satisfying task

Organizational characteristics
- Cohesive work group
- Low position power
- Formalization (roles, procedures)
- Inflexibility (rules, policies)
- Dispersed employee work sites

Consider a time when you participated in an ineffective or unsuccessful leadership event.

1. What employee characteristics hindered that process?
2. Describe the task characteristics that negatively affected the process.
3. Explain the organizational characteristics that stalled change.

Think of an example of when you have experienced effective or successful leadership.

1. What employee characteristics contributed to the success of the leadership process?
2. Identify and describe the task characteristics that enhanced the organization event.
3. Express the organizational characteristics that contributed to the overall success.

▋REFERENCES

Ayman, R., Chemers, M. M., & Fiedler, F. E. (1995). The contingency model of leadership effectiveness: Its levels of analysis. *Leadership Quarterly, 6*(2), 147–167.

Blanchard, K. H. (1985). *SLII: A situational approach to managing people.* Escondido, CA: Blanchard Training and Development.

Blank, W., Weitzel, J. R., & Green, S. G. (1990). A test of the situational leadership theory. *Personnel Psychology, 43*(3), 579–597.

Crouch, A., & Yetton, P. (1987). Manager behavior, leadership style, and subordinate performance: An empirical extension of the Vroom–Yetton Conflict Rule. *Organizational Behavior and Human Decision Processes, 39*(3), 384–396.

Dionne, S. D., Yammarino, F. J., Howell, J. P., & Villa, J. (2005). Theoretical letters: Substitutes for leadership, or not. *Leadership Quarterly, 16*(1), 169–193.

Fernandez, C. F., & Vecchio, R. P. (1997). Situational leadership theory revisited: A test of an across-jobs perspective. *Leadership Quarterly, 8*(1), 67–84.

Fiedler, F. E. (1964). A contingency model of leadership effectiveness. In L. Berkowitz (Ed.), *Advances in experimental social psychology.* New York, NY: Academic Press.

Fiedler, F. E. (1967). *A theory of leadership effectiveness.* New York, NY: McGraw-Hill.

Fiedler, F. E. (1971). Validation and extension of the contingency model of leadership effectiveness: A review of empirical findings. *Psychological Bulletin, 76*(2), 128–148.

Fiedler, F. E. (1978). The contingency model and the dynamics of the leadership process. In L. Berkowitz (Ed.), *Advances in experimental social psychology.* New York, NY: Academic Press.

Fiedler, F. E., & Chemers, M. M. (1982). *Improving leadership effectiveness: The leader match concept* (2nd ed.). New York, NY: John Wiley.

Fiedler, F. E., & Garcia, J. E. (1987). *New approaches to effective leadership: Cognitive resources and organizational performance.* New York, NY: Wiley.

Field, R. H. G. (1979). A critique of the Vroom–Yetton contingency model of leadership behavior. *Academy of Management Review, 4,* 249–257.

Graeff, C. L. (1983). The situational leadership theory: A critical view. *Academy of Management Review, 8,* 285–291.

Graeff, C. L. (1997). Evolution of situational leadership theory: A critical review. *Leadership Quarterly, 8*(2), 153–170.

Hersey, P., & Blanchard, K. (1982). *Management of organizational behavior: Utilizing human resources* (4th ed.). Englewood Cliffs, NJ: Prentice Hall.

Hersey, P., & Blanchard, K. H. (1993). *Management of organizational behavior: Utilizing human resources* (6th ed.). Englewood Cliffs, NJ: Prentice Hall.

House, R. J. (1971). A path-goal theory of leadership effectiveness. *Administrative Science Quarterly, 16,* 321–339.

House, R. J., & Mitchell, T. R. (1974). Path-goal theory of leadership. *Journal of Contemporary Business, 3*(4), 81–97.

Howell, J. P., Bowen, D. E., Dorfman, P. W., Kerr, S., & Podsakoff, P. M. (1990). Substitutes for leadership: Effective alternatives to ineffective leadership. *Organizational Dynamics, 19*(1), 21–38.

Jago, A. G. (1978). Configural cue utilization in implicit models of leader behavior. *Organizational Behavior and Human Performance, 22,* 474–496.

Jago, A. G., & Vroom, V. H. (1980). An evaluation of two alternatives to the Vroom/Yetton normative model. *Academy of Management Journal, 23,* 347–355.

Jermier, J. M. (1996). The path-goal theory of leadership: A subtextual analysis. *Leadership Quarterly, 7*(3), 311–316.

Kennedy, J. K., Jr. (1982). Middle LPC leaders and the contingency model of leadership effectiveness. *Organizational Behavior and Human Performance, 30*, 1–14.

Kerr, S., & Jermier, J. M. (1978). Substitutes for leadership: Their meaning and measurement. *Organizational Behavior and Human Performance, 22*, 375–403.

Northouse, P. (2007). *Leadership: Theory and practice* (4th ed.). Thousand Oaks, CA: Sage.

Northouse, P. (2010). *Leadership: Theory and practice* (5th ed.). Thousand Oaks, CA: Sage.

Peters, L. H., Hartke, D. D., & Pohlmann, J. T. (1985). Fiedler's contingency theory of leadership: An application of the meta-analysis procedures. *Psychological Bulletin, 97*(2), 274–285.

Podsakoff, P. M., & MacKenzie, S. B. (1997). Kerr and Jermier's substitutes for leadership model: Background, empirical assessment and suggestions for future research. *Leadership Quarterly, 8*(2), 117–125.

Podsakoff, P. M., MacKenzie, S. B., Ahearne, M., & Bommer, W. H. (1995). Searching for a needle in a haystack: Trying to identify the illusive moderators of leadership behaviors. *Journal of Management, 21*, 423–470.

Podsakoff, P. M., MacKenzie, S. B., & Bommer, W. H. (1996). Meta-analysis for the relationships between Kerr and Jermier's substitutes for leadership and employee job attitudes, role perceptions, and performance. *Journal of Applied Psychology, 81*(4), 380–399.

Podsakoff, P. M., MacKenzie, S. B., & Fetter, R. (1993). Substitutes for leadership and management of professionals. *Leadership Quarterly, 4*(1), 1–44.

Schriesheim, C. A., & Kerr, S. (1977). R.I.P. LPC: A response to Fiedler. In J. G. Hunt & L. L. Larson (Eds.), *Leadership: The cutting edge* (pp. 51–56). Carbondale,: Southern Illinois University Press.

Schriesheim, C. A., Tepper, B. J., & Tetrault, L. A. (1994). Least preferred co-worker score, situational control, and leadership effectiveness: A meta-analysis of contingency model performance predictions. *Journal of Applied Psychology, 79*(4), 561–573.

Shiflett, S. C. (1973). The contingency model of leadership effectiveness: Some implications of its statistical and methodological properties. *Behavioral Science, 18*(6), 429–440.

Stogdill, R., & Coons, A. (Eds.). (1957). *Leader behavior: Its description and measurement* (Research Monograph No. 88). Columbus: Ohio State University, Bureau of Business.

Strube, M. J., & Garcia, J. E. (1981). A meta-analytic investigation of Fiedler's contingency model of leadership effectiveness. *Psychological Bulletin, 90*(2), 307–321.

Thompson, G., & Vecchio, R. P. (2009). Situational leadership theory: A test of three versions. *Leadership Quarterly, 20*, 837–848.

Tjosvold, D., Wedley, W. C., Field, R. H. G. (1986). Constructive controversy, the Vroom–Yetton model, and managerial decision-making. *Journal of Occupational Behavior, 7*(2), 125–138.

Vecchio, R. P. (1987). Situational leadership theory: An examination of a prescriptive theory. *Journal of Applied Psychology, 72*(3), 444–451.

Vecchio, R. P., & Boatwright, K. J. (2002). Preferences for idealized style of supervision. *Leadership Quarterly, 13*, 327–342.

Vroom, V. H., & Jago, A. G. (1978). On the validity of the Vroom–Yetton model. *Journal of Applied Psychology, 63*(2), 151–162.

Vroom, V. H., & Jago, A. G. (1988). *The new leadership: Managing participation in organizations.* Englewood Cliffs, NJ: Prentice Hall.

Vroom, V. H., & Jago, A. G. (2007). The role of situation in leadership. *American Psychologist, 62*(1), 17–24.

Vroom, V. H., & Yetton, P. W. (1973). *Leadership and decision-making.* Pittsburgh, PA: University of Pittsburgh Press.

Williams, M. L., Podsakoff, P. M., Todor, W. D., Huber, V. L, Howell, J., & Dorfman, P. W. (1988). A preliminary analysis of construct validity of Kerr and Jermier's substitutes for leadership scales. *Journal of Occupational Psychology, 61*, 307–333.

Wofford, J. C., & Liska, L. Z. (1993). Path-goal theories of leadership: A meta-analysis. *Journal of Management, 19*(4), 857–876.

Yukl, G. (2010). *Leadership in organizations* (7th ed.). Upper Saddle River, NJ: Prentice Hall.

6

Contemporary Theories of Leadership

Brent J. Goertzen

A leader's role is to raise people's aspirations for what they can become and to release their energies so they will try to get there.

David Gergen, director of the Center for Public Leadership,
Harvard Kennedy School (from *http://www.leadershipnow.com*)

INTRODUCTION

The publication in 1978 of *Leadership*, James MacGregor Burns's bestselling book on political leadership, marked a major transition in the development of leadership theory. Much of the research in leadership since then has been largely influenced by his definition of "transforming leadership." Burns was the first to conceptualize leadership as a social process that involves both leaders and followers interacting and working together to achieve common interests and mutually defined ends. His theory clearly elevated the significance of followers and the leader–follower relationship in the leadership equation.

This chapter reviews Burns's transforming leadership theory and subsequent research that emerged as a result of his perspective. Also described are other contemporary leadership theories that emphasize the importance of the followers' role in leadership, such as the postindustrial paradigm of leadership, leader–member exchange (LMX) theory, followership, and servant leadership.

TRANSFORMING LEADERSHIP AND TRANSFORMATIONAL LEADERSHIP

Transforming Leadership

Burns (1978) is credited with revolutionizing scholars' and practitioners' view of leadership. Burns defined transforming leadership as occurring when "one or more persons engage with others in such a way that leaders and followers raise one another to higher levels of motivation and morality" (p. 20). Although initially starting out separate (and perhaps even unrelated), the purposes of both leaders and followers become fused. Leaders play a major role in shaping the relationship with followers. Burns believed that leaders are commonly more "skillful in evaluating followers' motives, anticipating their responses to an initiative, and estimating their power bases, than the reverse" (p. 20).

Transforming leadership has an elevating effect on both the leader and the led because it raises the level of human conduct and interaction. In the end, transforming leadership is a moral process because leaders engage with followers based on shared motives, values, and goals. Transforming leadership contrasts with transactional leadership, whereby the leadership relationship is limited to the leader's ability to appeal to followers' self-interest for the purpose of an exchange of valued things.

Burns asserts that only followers can ultimately define their true needs. This implies that followers must maintain freedom of choice between real alternatives. Transforming leaders operate at the highest stages of moral development. Burns (1978) asserted that transforming leaders are "guided by near-universal ethical principles of justice such as equality of human rights and respect of individual dignity" (p. 42).

Nonetheless, transforming leadership is grounded in conflict. Conflict is often compelling, because it galvanizes and motivates people. Leaders do not shun conflict; they embrace it by both shaping and mediating conflict. Leaders are able to discern signs of dissatisfaction among followers and take the initiative to make connections with followers. The power in transforming leadership comes by recognizing the varying needs and motives of potential followers and elevating them to transcend personal self-interests. Followers are mobilized by leaders' ability to appeal to and strengthen those motives through word and action.

Leadership Points to Ponder

Leadership is not magnetic personality that can just as well be a glib tongue. It is not "making friends and influencing people;" that is flattery. Leadership is lifting a person's vision to higher sights; the raising of a person's performance to a higher standard, the building of a personality beyond its normal limitations.

Peter F. Drucker (*from http://thinkexist.com*)

Transformational Leadership

Bass (1985, 1996) built upon Burns's (1978) original ideas of transforming leadership. He began empirically examining the theory and calling his revised theory "transformational leadership." These terms may seem nearly identical. However, there is an important distinction in that, whereas Burns's theory focuses more on social reform by moral elevation of followers' values and needs, Bass's transformational leadership focuses more on attaining practical organizational objectives (Yukl 2010).

Bass asserted that leaders demonstrating transformational leadership typically engage in several categories of behaviors. These behaviors typically enhance follower motivation and performance.

According to Bass (1985), transformational leaders are able to achieve three things: (1) make followers aware of the importance of task outcomes, (2) induce followers to transcend personal interest for the sake of the team or organization, and (3) move followers toward higher-order needs.

As a result, followers feel more confidence in the leader and report feeling greater trust, admiration, loyalty, and respect, especially when they are motivated to do more than they originally expected. Although numerous dimensions of transformational leader behaviors have been theorized and researched, it is commonly accepted that transformational leader behaviors comprise four categories: (1) idealized influence, (2) individualized consideration, (3) inspirational motivation, and (4) intellectual stimulation (Bass, 1997).

Transactional leadership behaviors refer to activities that help clarify expectations for direct reports, help direct reports achieve desired rewards and avoid punishments, and help facilitate desired outcomes (Avolio & Bass, 1988). Transactional leader behaviors commonly comprise three categories: (1) contingent reward, (2) management by exception—active, and (3) management by exception—passive.

Although transformational and transactional leader behaviors are distinct, they are not necessarily mutually exclusive. Effective leaders, Bass asserted, make use of both types of leadership. Whereas transformational leader behaviors enlist enthusiasm and commitment, transactional leadership behaviors achieve compliance with leader requests.

Recent versions of transformational and transactional theory include a third category of leadership: laissez-faire. This category represents an absence of effective leadership and describes the type of leader who is passive or indifferent to direct reports. Taken together, the three meta-categories (transformational, transactional, and laissez-faire) are sometimes called the Full Range Leadership model (Avolio, 1999; see **TABLE 6-1**).

Transformational and transactional leadership constitute the most widely researched models of leadership. They have been extensively studied in many different organizational contexts (e.g., corporations, militaries,

Table 6-1 Full Range Leadership Model

Transformational leadership	
Idealized influence	Leaders serve as outstanding role models for their followers. They display conviction, emphasize important personal values, and connect those values with organizational goals and ethical consequences of decisions.
Inspirational motivation	Leaders articulate an appealing vision of the future and challenge followers' high standards and high expectations. Leaders provide encouragement, optimism, and purpose for what needs to be done.
Intellectual stimulation	Leaders question old assumptions and stimulate new perspectives and innovative ways of doing things. They encourage followers to think creatively to address current and future challenges.
Individualized consideration	Leaders provide a supportive environment and carefully listen to followers' needs. Leaders also advise, teach, or coach their followers with the intention of advancing follower development.
Transactional leadership	
Contingent reward	Leaders offer followers rewards in exchange for desired efforts. Behaviors in this category revolve around clarifying expectations and exchanging promises.
Management by exception–active	Leaders observe follower behavior and take corrective action when followers deviate from expected performance.
Management by exception–passive	Leaders choose not to, or fail to, intervene until a problem becomes serious. In essence, leaders do not intervene until a problem is brought to their attention.
Laissez-faire leadership (nonleadership)	
Laissez-faire leadership	Leaders avoid accepting responsibility and delay or even fail to follow up on requests. This type of leader behavior also includes little or no effort to address followers' needs. It is essentially an absence of leadership.

Sources: Adapted from Bass (1997) and Northouse (2007).

government agencies, schools, and universities; Lowe, Kroeck, Sivasubramaniam, 1996) and cultures (e.g., the United States, Mexico, China, Japan, Indonesia, and Germany; Bass, 1997).

Transformational leadership is not limited to the upper echelons of organizations. Lowe and coauthors (1996) examined 23 published and unpublished studies examining transformational and transactional leadership. They found that leaders demonstrating transformational leader behaviors were more effective than those only demonstrating transactional leadership. Furthermore, they found that transformational leader behaviors were more common in public organizations compared to private organizations as perceived by the leaders' direct reports. The study also reported that leaders at lower levels of organizational hierarchy were more likely

to demonstrate transformational leader behaviors compared to executives holding higher-level positions. In addition, transformational leadership has been related to objective measures, such as financial performance (Rowold & Heinitz, 2007), sales performance (Yammarino & Dubinsky, 1994), and percent of goals met (Howell & Avolio, 1993).

Extensive research has been conducted examining the effect of transformational leader behaviors on followers and organizational outcomes. For example, Organ, Podsakoff, and MacKenzie (2006) found that transformational leader behaviors effected organizational citizenship behaviors among employees. Organizational citizenship behaviors are discretionary behaviors that are outside normal "in-role" job functions. In the aggregate, they promote effective organizational functioning (Organ,

1988). Organ and coauthors (2006) reported that transformational leadership directly influenced employee "altruism" citizenship behaviors. However, they also found that transformational leader behaviors directly affect employees' trust in their leader, which in turn also enhances employees' willingness to engage in other citizenship behaviors, such as "sportsmanship," "civic virtue," and "conscientiousness."

Other studies explained the impact of transformational leader behaviors on organizational outcomes differently. One study found that transformational leader behaviors directly affect employee "psychological capital" (Gooty, Gavin, Johnson, Frazier, & Snow, 2009). Positive psychological capital refers to positive-oriented human resource strengths and psychological capacities that improve the workplace (Luthans, 2002). These capacities include the dimensions of hope, self-efficacy, resiliency, and optimism. Psychological capital then increases employees' willingness to improve job performance and organizational citizenship behaviors directed at individuals and the organization (Gooty et al., 2009).

Bass (1997) reviewed literature that examined transformational leadership across cultures. He reported that although the mean and correlation strength may vary, the general pattern of the relationships between the transformational leader dimensions on measured outcomes (e.g., leader effectiveness, satisfaction, and extra effort) is the same.

However, there may be cultural contingencies on how each of the categories of transformational leader behaviors may be demonstrated. Yokochi (1989) reported that in a collectivist culture, such as Japan, there is an expectation that leaders will use individualized consideration. There is a mutual moral obligation between leaders and followers. Leaders are expected to help employees prepare for a career and counsel them about personal problems, and followers reciprocate with unquestioning loyalty and obedience. Additionally, Bass (1997) reported on other studies conducted across cultures that asked participants to describe their prototypical leaders. Avolio and Bass (1990) conducted extensive leadership development programs across the globe (e.g., Canada, Italy, Israel, Sweden, and Austria) and found that when individuals describe their ideal leaders, they commonly express transformational leadership qualities compared to transactional leadership qualities.

RELATIONAL LEADERSHIP

Leader–Member Exchange

Original studies of LMX theory asserted that managers develop differentiated relationships with direct reports within their organizations. According to the theory, managers develop high-quality relationships with only a few, high-trust direct reports. Managers reporting high-quality relationships (in-groups) characterize the exchange with high mutual respect, trust, and obligation on one end of a continuum. Low-quality relationships (out-groups), at the other end of the spectrum, are characterized by a relatively low degree of mutual respect, trust, and obligation (Dansereau, Graen, & Haga, 1975). This theory was originally labeled "vertical dyad linkage" because it focused on the reciprocal influence of managers and their direct reports within vertical dyads whereby one has direct authority over another (Yukl, 2010). There are tremendous advantages for direct reports who establish high-quality relationships. They tend to receive more desirable tasks assignments; are delegated greater authority; receive greater tangible rewards (e.g., pay increases); and receive greater approval and support.

Scholars assert that the manager–direct report relationship develops in a three-stage process described as a "life cycle model" (Graen & Uhl-Bien, 1995). The "stranger" stage begins when leaders and members first come together. This relationship is purely contractual in nature, whereby leaders provide members with what they need, and members perform prescribed work activities. In the "acquaintance" phase, the second of the life cycle stages, there is an increase in social exchanges. The relationship begins to transcend formal job requirements as leaders and members share greater information on a personal level, in addition to the work level. The third and final phase is described as a "mature partnership." These exchanges are highly developed and characterized by a mutual sense of trust, respect, and obligation. Participants in such relationships can count on one another for loyalty and support. How a dyad advances through each of these stages varies. Some dyads may not progress past the "stranger" phase and may maintain only the contractually based relationship. Others may rapidly progress to the "partnership" phase and achieve the tremendous advantages of a mature relationship.

LMX theory is one of the most widely studied leadership models. Gerstner and Day (1997) conducted a review of all published research on LMX and reported that high-quality LMX was positively related to such variables as performance ratings, objective performance, satisfaction with supervisor, overall satisfaction, organizational commitment, and role clarity. It was also positively related to organizational citizenship behaviors (Ilies, Nahrgang, & Morgeson, 2007). Low-quality LMX proved to be positively related to such variables as role conflict and turnover intentions.

There are many factors that influence the development of high-quality LMX. Research indicates that greater demographic similarity between the manager and direct reports, such as gender (Duchon, Green, & Taber, 1986; Green, Anderson, & Shivers, 1996), personality (Burns, 1995; Deluga, 1998), and attitudes (Dose, 1999; Steiner, 1988), were positively related to high-quality LMX. Other research focused on leader characteristics, such as attitudes, perceptions, and behavior, in the LMX relationship. For example, leader qualities, such as trust-building behavior (Deluga, 1994) and delegation (Bauer & Green, 1996), leader self-efficacy, and optimism (Murphy & Ensher, 1999) were positively related to LMX quality. Additional studies found that member characteristics, such as extraversion (Phillips & Bedeian, 1994), locus of control (Kinicki & Vecchio, 1994), self-efficacy (Murphy & Ensher, 1999), ingratiation (Deluga & Perry, 1994; Wayne, Liden, & Sparrowe, 1994), "in-role" behavior (Basu & Green, 1995), and subordinate performance (Basu & Green, 1995; Liden, Wayne, & Stilwell, 1993) were positively related to LMX quality. Finally, research examined the role of situational variables in the development of LMX. Perceived organizational support was positively related to high-quality LMX (Wayne, Shore, & Liden, 1997). Unit size was negatively related to high-quality LMX (Green et al., 1996). This means that the larger the departmental unit, the less likely leaders were to develop high-quality LMX relationships.

Leadership Points to Ponder

The single biggest way to impact an organization is to focus on leadership development. There is almost no limit to the potential of an organization that recruits good people, raises them up as leaders and continually develops them.

John C. Maxwell
The 17 Indisputable Laws of Teamwork (2001, p. 185)

People who have studied LMX have sought to assist managers in developing high-quality relationships with all members (Graen & Uhl-Bien, 1995). Expanding high-quality LMX beyond the typical select few who develop naturally provides two valuable benefits. First, it increases the perception of fairness among members and decreases suspicions of favoritism. Second, it increases the potential for "effective leadership and expanded organizational capability" (p. 229). Realistically, managers still develop differing relationships with their direct reports. Although theoretical models propose potential organizational (e.g., organizational culture and organizational structure), group (e.g., composition and size), and individual (e.g., leadership style and employees' desire for a high-quality relationship) antecedents to LMX differentiation and potential outcomes (Henderson, Liden, Glibkowski, & Chaudhry, 2009), further research is required to understand how these many different elements affect the development of LMX differentiation.

It is important to note that nearly all of the theory development and research examining LMX quality has been performed with the assumption of hierarchical relationships based on formal authority and reporting structures. Research is beginning to integrate both formally structured and informal relationships. Sparrowe and Liden (1997) theorized that leaders' and members' informal social networks affect the quality of LMX. Each is able to incorporate the other, through introductions and referrals, to their respective network of trusted contacts. As result, the added relational resources were theorized to enhance the work-related outcomes of the dyad members. Further, Balkundi, and Kilduff (2005) asserted that the range of one's social network across organizational boundaries will enhance personal benefits and organizational outcomes.

Research supports the notion that the breadth of one's informal social network positively affects LMX quality when the other member of the dyad is frequently sought for advice (Goodwin, Bowler, & Whittington, 2008). This indicates that leaders also recognize the value of members' social networks to the workings of the organization. Additionally, group leaders who were well connected in a friendship network of their peers at the same level in the organization outperformed their peers who were not as highly connected (Mehra, Dixon, Brass, & Robertson, 2006). This was likely because highly connected leaders have "better and faster access to information, advice and support" (p. 74).

Relational leadership is another emerging view of leadership that focuses on processes, not on persons, by which "leadership is produced and enabled" (Uhl-Bien, 2006). Relational leadership theory is defined as "a social influence process through which emergent conditions (i.e., evolving social order) and change (i.e., new values, attitudes, approaches, behaviors, ideologies, etc.) are constructed and produced" (p. 668). It assumes that leadership can occur in any direction. From this perspective, "it is possible to see relationships other than those built from hierarchy . . . and to envision transformational phenomenon where the social change process occurs well outside the normal assumptions of command and control (Murrell, 1997, p. 39).

Although the knowledge gained from these studies and insights developed from theoretical models proves fruitful for leader–member relationships in the context of organizations, the understanding of leader–member relationships based on informal networks and other relationships that transcend organizations in community-level leadership initiatives is severely limited. One can draw inferences from the current LMX literature and other relational leadership theory, but further research is required to more comprehensively understand the process of how relationships develop and their role in the leadership process.

POST INDUSTRIAL LEADERSHIP

Joseph Rost (1993) is credited with shifting scholars' focus from what he described as the industrial paradigm of leadership theory to the postindustrial paradigm. The subject of leadership did not exist before the 1890s, and the study of leadership has been a predominantly twentieth-century phenomena (Rost, 1997). Since that time, the basic ideas of leadership, in his view, had not changed much. He sharply criticized the popular assumptions about leadership at the time, which he described as (1) leadership is what great people do, (2) leadership and management are interchangeable, and (3) the terms "leadership" and "leader" are synonymous.

The concept of leadership in the industrial paradigm was bound up with what leaders do; the assumption was that no one else mattered. Therefore, followers had nothing to do with leadership and were typically perceived as being passive, submissive, and directed. After conducting an exhaustive review of leadership theory and research, Rost summarized the industrial paradigm definition of leadership as: "great men and women with certain preferred traits influencing followers to do what the leaders wish in order to achieve group/organizational goals that reflect excellence defined as some kind of higher-order effectiveness" (Rost, 1993, p. 180).

Rost contrasted the industrial paradigm of leadership with the radically different approach in the postindustrial age, which characterized leadership as relationship-based and focused on the noncoercive interaction of leaders and followers who develop common interests. Based on this perspective, Rost redefined leadership as "an influence relationship among leaders and followers who intend real changes that reflect their mutual purposes" (Rost, 1993, p. 102). There are four critical elements that comprise this definition of leadership, and each component is essential in understanding the postindustrial perspective: (1) the relationship is based on influence, (2) leaders and followers are participants in this relationship, (3) leaders and followers intend real changes, and (4) leaders and followers develop mutual purposes.

Leadership Points to Ponder

You must unite your constituents around a common cause and connect with them as human beings.

James Kouzes and Barry Posner
(from *http://www.youreffectiveleadership.com*)

Relationships Based on Influence

A leadership relationship must be based on influence, which is characterized as a process of using persuasion to affect other people. Although persuasion is largely composed of rational discourse, it may also include other aspects of "power resources," such as content of the message, purpose, symbolic interaction, perception, and motivation. Influence relationships are multidirectional, meaning they involve interactions that are vertical, horizontal, diagonal, and circular. This implies that anyone can be a leader or a follower, because leaders persuade followers and followers influence leaders. In the postindustrial paradigm, leaders and followers can actually switch places. Furthermore, relationships based on influence are inherently noncoercive. Coercion is antithetical to leadership because, according to Rost, it relies on authority or a power relationship that is dictatorial. Rost (1993) described dictatorial relationships as using people as objects, not as persons. As such, dictatorial relationships keep people in subservient roles. Freedom is necessary in influence relationships.

Leaders and Followers Are Participants

Leadership is a social process; therefore, leaders interact with other people. In the postindustrial paradigm, followers are no longer viewed as "the sweaty masses" or willing to let other people control their lives. Rather, followers must be active participants in the leadership process. Followers may fall anywhere on the continuum of the level of activity, but the important point is their willingness to be involved in the process and engage their power resources to influence other people. According to Rost (1993), followers do not "do followership." Rather, the interactions between leaders and followers comprise the leadership relationship. This does not mean that leaders and followers are equal in this relationship. Typically, leaders have more influence because they are willing to share (or perhaps even risk) more power resources than followers. However, there may be times when followers exert more influence in the relationship, particularly when they seize the initiative and drive the purposes in the relationship.

Participants Intend Real Change

There are two critical terms in this component of Rost's definition of leadership: intend and real. "Intend" indicates that leaders and followers are purposeful and desire certain changes in an organization or society. Because persons typically evaluate others' intentions by their words and deeds, intention must be demonstrated by action. The word "real" means that the purposes intended by leaders and followers must be significant and transforming. The postindustrial definition of leadership does not require participants to produce the changes for leadership to occur. Whereas intended changes are in the present and changes actually take place in the future (if at all), Rost's definition focuses more on the leadership process than the actual product or outcomes of the process. "A relationship wherein leaders and followers intend real changes but are unsuccessful or ineffective, or achieve only minimum changes, is still leadership" (Rost, 1993, p. 116).

Changes Reflect Mutual Interests

The final component of the postindustrial paradigm of leadership focuses on mutual purposes. For purposes to be mutual, they cannot rely solely on what leaders want or only on what the followers want. These mutual purposes emerge only through repeated and numerous interactions between leaders and followers. Rost carefully chooses the term "purposes" rather than "goals" because purposes are generally considered broader and more holistic and more closely related to the terms "vision" or "mission." Through noncoercive influence relationships, leaders and followers come to agreement and forge common interests and mutual purposes (Rost, 1997).

Proponents of the postindustrial paradigm of leadership also criticize leadership models purporting to view leadership as a social process, such as theories that focus on the dyadic relationship (e.g., LMX) between managers and their direct reports (Barker, 1997).

> *This concept of leadership is founded in the feudal touchstone of citizenship: one's relationship with one's king. This relationship implies several assumptions: (a) that the king deserves allegiance by virtue of rank, (b) that there is a natural, hierarchical difference in status, intelligence, and ability, (c) and that the subject's role is to serve the king's wishes. (Barker, 1997, p. 350)*

Barker differentiated leadership as a social relationship and leadership as a social process. He asserted that leadership as a social relationship tends to be contractual in nature based on role expectations. However, leadership as a social process, which includes social relationships, is much broader in that it provides flexibility in the creation of new relationships, roles, and expectations where none may have existed. These relationships look far beyond hierarchical, organizational structures to include informal social networks (within and outside an organizational context) and intraorganizational relationships, among other types of relationships not based on formal authority connections. Barker likened the leadership process to a river:

> *Contained by its bed (the culture), it can be said to be flowing in one direction, yet, upon close examination, parts of it flow sideways, in circles, or even backwards relative to the overall direction. It is constantly changing in speed and strength, and even reshapes its*

own container. Under certain conditions, it is very unified in direction and very powerful; under other conditions it may be weak or may flow in many directions at once. (Barker, 1997, p. 352)

The postindustrial paradigm of leadership developed by Rost and others has tremendous intuitive and practical appeal and offers valuable potential for leadership education. Effective leadership curricula ought to include three broad categories: (1) evolution of social change and development, (2) processes influencing social change, and (3) dynamics of human nature in change processes (Rost & Barker, 2000).

Unfortunately, scholars have been slow to embrace the postindustrial paradigm of leadership. One recent study examined historical records to describe the context and process of the Nez Perce leadership council as an exemplar of the paradigm (Humphreys, Ingram, Kernek, & Sadler, 2007). However, few have empirically investigated it to confirm or disprove the veracity of its components. Perhaps this perspective of leadership does not lend itself well to rational, scientific inquiry. If leadership is defined as a social process (as identified by Barker), one must view relationships and their potential creation and dissolution as a rather nebulous construct. This causes tremendous challenges for scholars applying the scientific method to not only describe its nature, but also predict potential antecedents and outcomes.

FOLLOWERSHIP

To raise the importance of the role of followers in the leadership process, researchers have proposed several theories that describe the leadership capacities of followers. This is not to minimize the relevance of leaders, but rather to enhance the understanding of the vital role that followers play in the leadership relationship.

Effective Followership

Kelley (1988) asserted that what differentiated effective from ineffective followers were their enthusiasm, intelligence, and self-reliant participation. He described a two-dimensional model that explained follower behavior. The first dimension describes the degree to which followers exercise independent and critical thinking. The second ranks them on a passive–active scale. Based on the two dimensions, four categories of followers emerge (**FIGURE 6-1**).

Sheep, according to Kelley, are passive and are generally unwilling to accept responsibility. They typically complete tasks given to them but rarely demonstrate initiative beyond those tasks. "Yes" people are more involved but are equally unwilling to demonstrate innovation or creativity. Alienated followers express critical and independent thinking but are passive in their roles; at some point, they were turned off. Although they rarely openly oppose the leader, they are often cynical and disgruntled. At the center of the diagram are survivors. They tend to adapt and survive change well but often live by the slogan "better safe than sorry." Effective followers, at the upper right quadrant of the diagram, effectively think for themselves in carrying out tasks and bring energy and enthusiasm while demonstrating initiative and assertiveness. Four qualities are shared by effective followers: (1) they manage themselves well; (2) they are committed to the organization or purpose outside themselves; (3) they build their competence; and (4) they are courageous, credible, and honest.

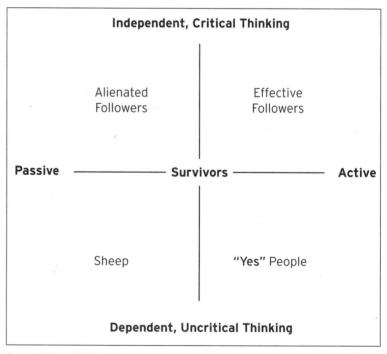

Source: Kelley (1998).

Figure 6-1 Follower behavior.

Effective followers tend to be actively involved in the life of the organization. They openly disagree with the leader and are not intimidated by hierarchy. Because they demonstrate initiative, they rarely need elaborate supervisory systems. Effective followers display commitment to a cause, product, or idea; however, they temper their loyalties to satisfy organizational needs.

Effective followers master important knowledge and skills necessary for their organization. These followers happily take on extra work that stretches their current capacities because they do not mind chancing failure. Further, effective followers establish themselves as credible and trustworthy and hold to ethical standards in which they believe.

Leadership Points to Ponder

The signs of outstanding leadership appear primarily among the followers. Are the followers reaching their potential? Are they learning? Serving? Do they achieve the required results? Do they change with grace? Manage conflict?

Max De Pree (from *Leadership is an Art,* 2004)

Courageous Followership

Challeff (1995) also asserted that "follower" is not a synonym for "subordinate." Followers are effective stewards for the organization and its resources. Challeff describes five dimensions of courage that are essential to effective followership:

1. Courage to assume responsibility: followers who discover and create new opportunities for themselves. They do not take a paternalistic view of their organization whereby they expect their supervisors to provide for their growth or permission to act.

2. Courage to serve: followers who are willing to work hard and serve their leader and organization. Effective followers display numerous behaviors in this dimension of courageous followership. For instance, followers can help the leader define and communicate the vision of the organization to all levels (Challeff, 2002). Courage to serve can also encompass behaviors intended to "conserve the leader's energy" by perhaps serving as a buffer and managing crises on the leader's behalf.

3. Courage to challenge: followers who engage in potential conflict as they voice their sense of what is right. Effective followers may risk rejection but nonetheless are willing to stand up for their beliefs. Although courageous followers value organizational harmony, they are willing to confront when individual or organizational activities violate the common purpose or integrity.

4. Courage to participate in transformation: followers who are involved in organizational transformation. Courageous followers may even serve as champions of organizational change, while still struggling with the discomfort and disequilibrium of the change process themselves.

5. Courage to take moral action: followers who know when to take a stand that is different from that of their leaders. This dimension of courage may put followers at risk because they may refuse a direct order, may seek to go above the leader's head, or may submit a resignation. Courageous followers are motivated by a higher purpose and are unwilling to compromise moral principles even in the face of tremendous risk to themselves.

Challeff described courageous followers as possessing tremendous power. Granted, followers do not possess formal power equal to that of leaders (1995). However, courageous followers appeal to other sources of power that are quite different from those of the leader. There is a wide range of followers' power:

- Power of purpose, common good
- Power of knowledge, skills, or resources
- Power of personal history, record of personal success in the organization
- Power of faith in self, integrity, commitment
- Power to speak the truth
- Power to set a standard that influences others
- Power to choose how to react in situations regardless of what is done or threatened
- Power to follow (or not)
- Power of relationships and networks
- Power to communicate through many channels
- Power to organize others
- Power to withdraw support

Numerous other conceptual models regarding effective followership have been published in the academic literature and popular press. Baker (2007) reviewed the various followership models and discovered that they shared four primary themes. First, followers and leaders are roles, not people with inherent characteristics. Most individuals, regardless of their positions in an organizational structure, have played the roles of both follower and leader in their organizations. Second, followers are active, not passive. This is contrary to popular views that followers are passive, obedient sheep. Demonstrating followership requires both parties (leaders and followers) to be active participants in the leader–follower relationship. Third, followers and leaders share a common purpose. Common purpose emerges out of an interdependent leader–follower relationship. Participants in followership remain committed to organizational goals. Finally, followership is built on the relational nature of both leaders and followers. The relationship is a two-way influence process. This collaborative partnership values the contributions of both leaders and followers.

Howell and Shamir (2005) contended that "understanding followers is as important as understanding leaders" (p. 110). Yukl (2010) rightly asserted that theories focusing almost exclusively on leaders or on followers are limiting, especially compared to more balanced explanations. Nonetheless, followership offers useful insights by describing qualities that are important for followers to be effectively engaged in the leadership process.

SERVANT LEADERSHIP

Greenleaf (1977) proposed the concept of servant leadership. For Greenleaf, the primary responsibility of leaders is to provide service to others. Spears (1995) asserted that the servant leader emphasizes "service to others, a holistic approach to work, a sense of community, and shared decision making power" (pp. 3–4). For the servant leader, taking care of other people's needs takes highest priority. Greenleaf (1977) described a series of questions that serve as a litmus test of the servant leader: "Do those served grow as persons? Do they, while being served, become healthier, wiser, freer, more autonomous, more likely themselves to become servants? And, what is the effect on the least privileged of society; will they benefit, or at least, not be further deprived?" (pp. 13–14).

Servant leadership, in essence, is a philosophic approach to life and work. Put differently, Spears (1995) stated, "at its core, servant-leadership is a long-term, transformational approach to life and work, in essence, a way of being that has the potential to create positive change throughout society" (p. 4). Servant leadership is a long-term pursuit of the improvement of corporate cultures and is not consistent with short-run profit motives (Giampetro-Meyer, Brown, Browne, & Kubasek, 1998).

Spears built on Greenleaf's original writing by identifying 10 characteristics of the servant leader.

1. Listening: The deep, heartfelt commitment to listening intently to others.
2. Empathy: Recognizing and accepting people for their special talents, gifts, and unique spirit.
3. Healing: People may have broken spirits or a variety of emotional hurts, thus an essential gift of the servant leader is not only to heal one's self, but also to assist in the healing of others.
4. Awareness: Refers primarily to self-awareness, which aides and strengthens the servant leader by providing an understanding of issues from a well-developed sense of ethics and values.
5. Persuasion: Servant leaders seek to convince rather than coerce and can be thought of as a "gentle persuasion" by challenging others to think of issues in different perspectives.
6. Conceptualization: The capacity to "dream great dreams." The servant leader is able to envision the future not only in the context of the individual, work group, or organization, but also within the context of the societal realm.
7. Foresight: The ability that enables servant leaders to glean lessons from the past, within the realities of the present, and understand potential consequences of future decisions.
8. Stewardship: The perspective that corporate institutions play a significant and vital role in affecting the greater good of society.
9. Commitment to growth of people: Every individual has an intrinsic worth beyond their contributions as workers. Servant leaders seek the holistic growth and development of others.
10. Building community: The servant leader takes advantage of opportunities to create community in the context of the given work institution.

Leadership Points to Ponder

We must be silent before we can listen.

We must listen before we can learn.

We must learn before we can prepare.

We must prepare before we can serve.

We must serve before we can lead.

William Arthur Ward (from *http://thinkexist.com*)

Graham (1991) compared and contrasted servant leadership with other popular theories of leadership to explain the moral gaps in the other leadership theories. "Weberian charismatic authority" refers to individuals who gain and maintain their authority by proving their powers to be a divinely inspired mission (Weber, 1978). The genuineness of charismatic leaders' authority rests on how well they provide for the well-being of followers. Charismatic authority often emerges from periods of tremendous crisis, such as great socioeconomic unrest, when traditional authorities fail to meet people's needs. Charismatic leaders offer a "divinely inspired" vision and perhaps even practical solutions with them in charge (Tucker, 1968).

Personal celebrity charisma is a slightly different version of charismatic leadership. House (1977) asserted that it required four personal characteristics: "dominance, self-confidence, need for influence, and a strong conviction in the moral righteousness of his or her beliefs" (p. 205). Leaders with personal celebrity charisma commonly occupy higher levels of organizations with greater visibility. Followers are more likely to attribute the "aura of magic" to those who are at greater organizational distance because, according to Katz and Kahn (1978), intimacy destroys the illusion. Followers of this type of leader often respond with adulation and emulation, but over time followers become addicted to passivity (Graham, 1991).

Transformational leadership incorporated some principles of charismatic leadership theory but added leader behaviors, such as individualized consideration and intellectual stimulation. These changes in leadership theory occurred because scholars began to recognize and value the contributions of followers by recognizing that subordinates (often labeled as "followers") were educated with the capacity for creativity. However, there is nothing in transformational leadership that says leaders should

serve the good of followers (Graham, 1991). Transformational leaders are typically more concerned with organizational goals.

Servant leadership, according to Graham (1991), restores the moral compass articulated by Burns's (1978) perspective of "transforming leadership." Burns asserted that effective (transforming) leaders focus on the ethical aspirations of both the leader and the led and stress end-values, such as liberty, justice, and equality. Servant leadership addresses this issue by focusing on the leader–follower relationship and on the ideal of service. Graham (1991) asserted, "leaders who not only listen to subordinates and other stakeholders, but allow themselves to be influenced by what they hear, are more powerful than those who rule by fiat" (p. 112). Servant leadership extends Bass's (1985, 1988) theory of transformational leadership in two ways: it recognizes the social responsibility in the call to serve, and it answers the question, Why should people grow even if they do not want to? (Graham, 1991). Greenleaf's (1977) claim that people should be served by someone who influences them to become wiser, freer, and more autonomous "is to say that it is in people's interest to change in those ways" (Graham, 1991, p. 113; **TABLE 6-2**).

Servant leadership may be effective leadership theory that possesses nearly universal cultural appeal. Servant leaders focus more on humility, the needs of others, and higher-order values, such as duty and social responsibility, than on self-interest. Humane orientation refers to the concern for the welfare of other people and willingness to sacrifice self-interest to help others (House, Hanges, Javidan, Dorfman, & Gupta, 2004). As such, Winston and Ryan (2008) persuasively argue that servant leadership is compatible with the humane-oriented culture that resonates with some African (Ubuntu, Harambee), East Asian (Taoist, Confucianism), Mediterranean (Jewish), and Indian (Hindu) cultures.

Unfortunately, servant leadership has limited empirical research to support its effectiveness. Yukl (2010) noted that much of the evidence for servant leadership is based on anecdotal accounts and case studies of leaders or organizations. Only recently have questionnaires been created (Barbuto & Wheeler, 2006; Liden, Wayne, Zhao, & Henderson, 2008); however, they are at the early stages of development.

The few empirical studies that have been published suggest that servant leadership may be a promising

Table 6-2 Comparison of "Charismatic" Leadership Models

	Weberian Charismatic Authority	Celebrity-Based Charisma	Transformational Leadership	Servant Leadership
Source of charisma	Divine gift	Personality; social distance	Leader training and skills	Humility, spiritual insight
Situational context	Socioeconomic distress of followers	Low self-esteem of followers	Unilateral (hierarchical) power	Relational (mutual) power
Nature of charismatic gift	Visionary solution to distress	Daring; dramatic flair; forcefulness; appealing vision	Vision for organization; adept at human resource management	Vision and practice of a way of life focused on service
Response of followers	Recognition of genuine divine gift	Adulation of and identification with leader	Heightened motivation; extra effort	Emulation of leader's service orientation
Consequences of charisma	Followers' material well-being improved	Codependent relationship with leader perpetuated	Leader or organizational goals met; personal development of followers	Autonomy and moral development of followers; enhancement of common good
Applicability to work organizations	No	Yes	Yes	Yes
Representative authors and concepts	Tucker; Weber	Conger & Kanungo; House; Howell's "personalized charisma"; Schiffer	Bass & associates; Bradford & Cohen; Howell's "socialized charisma"	Burns's "transforming leaders"; Greenleaf

Leadership Quarterly, 2(2), 107, Graham, Jill W. (1991) Servant leadership in organizations: Inspirational and moral. Reprinted with permission from Elsevier.

leadership perspective. Dimensions of servant leadership are related to positive outcomes in job performance, organizational commitment, and community commitment (Liden et al., 2008). In another study, elements of servant leadership were positively related to other organizational outcomes, such as extra effort, employee satisfaction, and organizational effectiveness (Barbuto & Wheeler, 2006). Nonetheless, further research is required to confirm the effectiveness of servant leadership.

SUMMARY

Burns revolutionized the understanding of effective leadership by conceptualizing it as transforming, a condition that occurs when "one or more persons engage with

others in such a way that leaders and followers raise one another to higher levels of motivation and morality" (1978, p. 20). This view lifts up the role of the follower to active participant in the leadership process. Followers are active in that they engage with leaders to develop mutual interests based on common values and needs.

The work of Bass and others refined Burns's concept of leadership and differentiated transformational leadership from transactional leadership. Transactional leadership refers to activities aimed at helping to clarify expectations and desired outcomes. It comprises categories of behaviors, such as contingent reward, management by exception—active, and management by exception—passive. Transformational leader behaviors, however, are intended to help instill confidence and enthusiasm in followers to rise above (transcend) what they believe they would normally be capable of doing. Categories of transformational leader behaviors include idealized influence, individualized consideration, inspirational motivation, and intellectual stimulation.

Rost strongly criticized much of the prior leadership theory and scholarship by characterizing it as largely developed from an industrial paradigm. He asserted that scholars and practitioners of leadership need to reconceptualize it for the postindustrial age in which we live. He defined the postindustrial paradigm of leadership as "an influence relationship among leaders and followers who intend real changes that reflect their mutual purposes" (1993, p. 102). Rost's paradigm comprises four critical elements: (1) leadership is based on influence (not coercion or authority); (2) leaders and followers are people in this relationship; (3) leaders and followers intend real change; and (4) leaders and followers develop mutual interests.

With the elevated status of the important role of followers, several models have sought to explain the specific roles of followers. According to Kelley (1988), effective followers manage themselves well, are committed to the organization or purposes outside themselves, build their own competence, and are credible and honest. Challeff (1995) also described the courage that effective followers must demonstrate. His model depicted effective followers as displaying the courage to assume responsibility, the courage to serve, the courage to challenge, the courage to participate in transformation, and the courage to take moral action.

Developed by Greenleaf, servant leadership is a model of leadership that describes leaders who are motivated primarily by providing service to others and taking care of other people's needs first. According to Greenleaf, the ultimate test of a servant leader is whether those being served were likely to "become healthier, wiser, freer, more autonomous, more likely themselves to become servants" (Greenleaf, 1977, pp. 13–14). Spears asserted that servant leadership requires "service to others, a holistic approach to work, a sense of community, and shared decision making power" (1995, pp. 3–4). Spears built on Greenleaf's original writing by identifying 10 characteristics of the servant leader: (1) listening, (2) empathy, (3) healing, (4) awareness, (5) persuasion, (6) conceptualization, (7) foresight, (8) stewardship, (9) commitment to growth of people, and (10) building community.

6

Wrap-Up

ACTIVITY

Transformational Leadership

Select a leader you consider to be highly effective. The person you select could be from your work or organization.

Describe the leader.

1. Explain how the leader is emotionally expressive.

2. Describe how clearly the leader articulates a vision for the future.

3. Detail how the leader communicates optimism and confidence in followers to achieve excellence.

4. Illustrate how the leader displays exceptional conceptual skills in approaching challenges in novel and unique ways.

5. Explain how the leader is able to draw out the best from the followers.

Describe the reaction of followers.

1. Elaborate on the followers' reaction to the leader.

2. Are followers likely to respect and admire the leader? Explain.

3. Does the leader instill pride in the followers? How does this occur?

4. Are followers more enthusiastic and eager for the work to be done? Explain.

5. Are the followers willing to exert extra effort for the leader?

6. Explain how the leader inspires innovative thinking to problems.

Leader–Member Relationships

Ask three employees in your organization (individuals who report directly to you) to complete the following survey regarding the quality of LMX (**FIGURE 6-2**). Answer the reflection questions.

1. Describe the highlights of your employees' perceptions regarding the LMX quality with you.

2. Which specific areas of your relationship with them could be improved?

3. What steps can you take to help improve the quality of LMX with your employees during the next month?

Affect							
1. I like my supervisor very much as a person.	0	1	2	3	4	5	6
2. My supervisor is the kind of person I would like to have as a friend.	0	1	2	3	4	5	6
3. My supervisor is a lot of fun to work with.	0	1	2	3	4	5	6
Loyalty							
4. My supervisor defends my work actions to a superior, even without complete knowledge of the issue in question.	0	1	2	3	4	5	6
5. My supervisor would come to my defense if I were "attacked" by others.	0	1	2	3	4	5	6
6. My supervisor would defend me to others in the organization if I made an honest mistake.	0	1	2	3	4	5	6
Contribution							
7. I do work for my supervisor that goes beyond what is specified in my job description.	0	1	2	3	4	5	6
8. I am willing to apply extra effort, beyond those normally required, to meet my supervisor's work goals.	0	1	2	3	4	5	6
9. I do not mind working my hardest for my supervisor.	0	1	2	3	4	5	6
Professional Respect							
10. I am impressed with my supervisor's knowledge of his/her job.	0	1	2	3	4	5	6
11. I respect my supervisor's knowledge of and competence on the job.	0	1	2	3	4	5	6
12. I admire my supervisor's professional skills.	0	1	2	3	4	5	6

Calculate a score for each of the four dimensions of LMX quality: strongly agree (6); moderately agree (5); somewhat agree (4); neutral (3); somewhat disagree (2); moderately disagree (1); strongly disagree (0). Consider the subtotal for each of the four dimensions.

Affect _____ out of 18

Loyalty _____ out of 18

Contribution _____ out of 18

Professional respect _____ out of 18

Source: Adapted from Liden & Maslyn (1998).

Figure 6-2 LMX–MDM Survey.

Servant Leadership

Watch the following clip from YouTube (http://www .youtube.com/watch?v=BHIKRmEaC6Y) and reflect on Tom Peters' perspective of servant leadership. What have you done in the last 24 hours to be of service to those around you? What will you do in the next 24 hours to be of service to those around you?

▐ REFERENCES

Avolio, B. J. (1999). *Full leadership development: Building the vital forces in organizations.* Thousand Oaks, CA: Sage.

Avolio, B. J., & Bass, B. M. (1988). Transformational leadership, charisma and beyond. In J. G. Hunt, H. R. Baliga, H. P. Dachler, & C. A. Schriesheim (Eds.), *Emerging leadership vistas* (pp. 29–50). Lexington, MA: Heath.

Avolio, B. J., & Bass, B. M. (1990). *The full range of leadership development: Basic/advanced manuals.* Binghamton, NY: Avolio/Bass and Associates.

Baker, S. D. (2007). Followership: The theoretical foundation of a contemporary construct. *Journal of Leadership & Organizational Studies, 14*(1), 50–60.

Balkundi, P., & Kilduff, M. (2005). The ties that lead: A social network approach to leadership. *Leadership Quarterly, 16,* 941–961.

Barbuto, J. E., & Wheeler, D. W. (2006). Scale development and construct clarification of servant leadership. *Group & Organizational Management, 31*(3), 300–326.

Barker, R. A. (1997). How can we train leaders if we do not know what leadership is? *Human Relations, 50*(4), 343–362.

Bass, B. M. (1985). *Leadership and performance: Beyond expectations.* New York, NY: Free Press.

Bass, B. M. (1988). Evolving perspectives on charismatic leadership. In J. A. Conger, R. N. Kanungo, & Associates (Eds.), *Charismatic leadership: The elusive factor in organizational effectiveness* (pp. 40–77). San Francisco, CA: Jossey-Bass.

Bass, B. M. (1996). *A new paradigm of leadership: An inquiry into transformational leadership.* Alexandria, VA: U.S. Army Research Institute for the Behavioral and Social Sciences.

Bass, B. M. (1997). Does transactional-transformational leadership paradigm transcend organizational and national boundaries? *American Psychologist, 52*(2), 130–139.

Basu, R., & Green, S. (1995). Subordinate performance, leader-subordinate compatibility, and exchange quality in leader-member dyads: A field study. *Journal of Applied Social Psychology, 25,* 77–92.

Bauer, T. N., & Green, S. G. (1986). Development of leader-member exchange: A longitudinal test. *Academy of Management Journal, 39*(6), 1538–1567.

Burns, J. L. Z. (1995). Prediction of leader-member exchange quality by Jungian personality type. *Dissertation Abstracts International.*

Burns, J. M. (1978). *Leadership.* New York, NY: Harper & Row Publishers.

Challeff, I. (1995). *The courageous follower: Standing up to and for our leaders.* San Francisco, CA: Berrett-Koehler.

Challeff, I. (2002). *The courageous follower: Standing up to and for our leaders* (2nd ed). San Francisco, CA: Berrett-Koehler.

Dansereau, F., Jr., Graen, G., & Haga, W. J. (1975). A vertical dyad linkage approach to leadership within formal organizations: A longitudinal investigation of the role-making approaches. *Organizational Behavior and Human Performance, 13,* 46–78.

Deluga, R. J. (1994). Supervisor trust building, leader-member exchange and organizational citizenship behavior. *Journal of Occupational and Organizational Psychology, 67,* 315–326.

Deluga, R. J. (1998). Leader-member exchange quality and effectiveness ratings. *Group and Organization Management, 23*(2), 189–216.

Deluga, R. J., & Perry, J. T. (1994). The role of subordinate performance and ingratiation in leader-member exchanges. *Group and Organization Management, 19*(1), 67–86.

Dose, J. J. (1999). The relationship between work values similarity and team-member and leader-member exchange relationships. *Group Dynamics: Theory, Research and Practice, 3*(1), 20–32.

Duchon, D., Green, S. G., & Taber, T. D. (1986). Vertical dyad linkage: A longitudinal assessment of antecedents, measures and consequences. *Journal of Applied Psychology, 71*(1), 56–60.

Gerstner, C. R., & Day, D. V. (1997). Meta-analytic review of leader-member exchange theory: Correlates and construct issues. *Journal of Applied Psychology, 82*(6), 827–844.

Giampetro-Meyer, A., Brown, T., Browne, M. N., & Kubasek, N. (1998). Do we really want more leaders in business? *Journal of Business Ethics, 17,* 1727–1736.

Goodwin, V. L., Bowler, W. M., & Whittington, J. L. (2008). A social network perspective on LMX relationships: Accounting for the instrumental value of leader and follower networks. *Journal of Management, 35*(4), 954–980.

Gooty, J., Gavin, M., Johnson, P. D., Frazier, M. L., & Snow, D. B. (2009). In the eyes of the beholder: Transformational leadership, positive psychological capital, and performance. *Journal of Leadership and Organizational Studies, 15*(4), 353–367.

Graen, G. B., & Uhl-Bien, M. (1995). Relationship-based approach to leadership: Development of leader-member exchange (LMX) theory of leadership over 25 years: Applying a multi-level multi-domain perspective. *Leadership Quarterly, 6,* 219–247.

Graham, J. W. (1991). Servant leadership in organizations: Inspirational and moral. *Leadership Quarterly, 2*(2), 105–119.

Green, S. G., Anderson, S. E., & Shivers, S. L. (1996). Demographic and organizational influences on leader-member exchange and related work attitudes. *Organizational Behavior and Human Decision Processes, 66*(2), 203–214.

Greenleaf, R. (1977). *Servant leadership.* New York, NY: Paulist Books.

Henderson, D. J., Liden, R. C., Glibkowski, B. C., & Chaudhry, A. (2009). LMX differentiation: A multi-level review and examination of its antecedents. *Leadership Quarterly, 20,* 517–534.

House, R. J. (1977). A 1976 theory of charismatic leadership. In J. G. Hunt & L. L. Larson (Eds.), *Leadership: The cutting edge* (pp. 189–207). Carbondale, IL: Southern Illinois University Press.

House, R., Hanges, P., Javidan, M., Dorfman, P., & Gupta, V. (Eds.). (2004). *Culture, leadership and organizations: The GLOBE study of 62 societies* (pp. 29–48). Thousand Oaks, CA: Sage.

Howell, J. M., & Avolio, B. J. (1993). Transformational leadership, transactional leadership, locus of control and support for innovation: Key predictors of consolidated business-unit performance. *Journal of Applied Psychology, 78,* 891–902.

Howell, J. M., & Shamir, B. (2005). The role of followers in the charismatic leadership process: Relationships and their consequences. *Academy of Management Review, 30,* 96–122.

Humphreys, J., Ingram, K., Kernek, C., & Sadler, T. (2007). The Nez Perce leadership council: A historical examination of post-industrial leadership. *Journal of Management History, 13*(2), 135–152.

Ilies, R., Nahrgang, J. D., & Morgeson, F. P. (2007). Leader-member exchange and citizenship behaviors: A meta-analysis. *Journal of Applied Psychology, 92*(1), 269–277.

Katz, D., & Kahn, R. L. (1978). *The social psychology of organizations* (2nd ed.). New York, NY: John Wiley & Sons.

Kelley, R. E. (1988). In praise of followers. *Harvard Business Review, 66,* 142–148.

Kinicki, A. J., & Vecchio, R. P. (1994). Influences of the quality of supervisor-subordinate relations: The role of time-pressure, organizational commitment, and locus of control. *Journal of Organizational Behavior, 15*(1), 75–82.

Liden, R. C., & Maslyn, J. M. (1998). Multidimensionality of leader–member exchange: An imperical assessment through scale development. *Journal of Management, 24:* 43–72.

Liden, R. C., Wayne, S. J., & Stilwell, D. (1993). A longitudinal study on the early development of leader-member exchanges. *Journal of Applied Psychology, 78*(4), 662–674.

Liden, R. C., Wayne, S. J., Zhao, H., & Henderson, D. (2008). Servant leadership: Development of a multidimensional measure and multi-level assessment. *Leadership Quarterly, 19,* 161–177.

Lowe, K. B., Kroeck K. G., & Sivasubramaniam N. (1996). Effectiveness correlates of transformational and transactional leadership: A meta-analytic review of the MLQ literature. *Leadership Quarterly, 7*(3), 385–425.

Luthans, F. (2002). Positive organizational behavior: Developing and managing psychological strengths. *Academy of Management Executive, 16,* 57–72.

Mehra, A., Dixon, A. L., Brass, D. J., & Robertson, B. (2006). The social network ties of group leaders:

implications for group performance and leader reputation. *Organization Science, 17*(1), 64–79.

Murphy, P. E. (1999). Character and virtue ethics in international marketing: An agenda for managers, researchers and educators. *Journal of Business Ethics, 18*, 107–124.

Murrell, K. L. (1997). Emergent theories of leadership for the next century: Towards relational concepts. *Organization Development Journal, 15*(3), 35–42.

Northouse, P. (2007). *Leadership: Theory and practice.* Thousand Oaks, CA: Sage Publications.

Organ, D. (1988). *Organizational citizenship behavior: The good soldier syndrome.* Lexington, MA: Lexington Books.

Organ, D. W., Podsakoff, P. M., & MacKenzie, S. B. (2006). *Organizational citizenship behaviors: Its nature, antecedents, and consequences.* Thousand Oaks, CA: Sage Publications.

Phillips, A. S., & Bedeian, A. G. (1994). Leader-follower exchange quality: The role of personal and interpersonal attributes. *Academy of Management Journal, 37*, 990–1001.

Rost, J. C. (1993). *Leadership for the 21st century.* New York, NY: Praeger.

Rost, J. C. (1997). Moving from industrial to relationship: A post-industrial paradigm of leadership. *Journal of Leadership Studies, 4*(4), 3–16.

Rost, J., & Barker, R. A. (2000). Leadership education in colleges: Toward a 21st century paradigm. *Journal of Leadership Studies, 7*(1), 3–12.

Rowold, J., & Heinitz, K. (2007). Transformational and charismatic leadership: Assessing the convergent, divergent and criterion validity of the MLQ and the CKS. *Leadership Quarterly, 18*, 121–133.

Sparrowe, R. T., & Liden, R. C. (1997). Process and structure in leader-member exchanges. *Academy of Management Review, 22*(2), 522–552.

Spears, L. C. (1995). *Reflections on leadership.* New York, NY: John Wiley & Sons.

Steiner, D. D. (1988). Value perceptions in leader-member exchange. *Journal of Social Psychology, 128*, 611–618.

Tucker, R. C. (1968). The theory of charismatic leadership. *Daedulus, 97*, 731–756.

Uhl-Bien, M. (2006). Relational leadership theory: Exploring the social processes of leadership and organizing. *Leadership Quarterly, 17*, 654–676.

Wayne, S. J., Liden, R. C., & Sparrowe, R. T. (1994). Developing leader-member exchanges: The influence of gender and ingratiation. *American Behavioral Scientist, 37*(5), 697–714.

Wayne, S. J., Shore, L. M., & Liden, R. C. (1997). Perceived organizational support and leader-member exchange: A social exchange perspective. *Academy of Management Journal, 40*(1), 82–111.

Weber, M. (1978). In G. Roth & C. Wittich (Eds.), *Economy and society: An outline of interpretive sociology.* Berkeley: University of California Press.

Winston, B. E., & Ryan, B. (2008). Servant leadership as a humane orientation: Using the GLOBE study construct of humane orientation to show that servant leadership is more global than western. *International Journal of Leadership Studies, 3*(2), 212–222.

Yammarino, F. J., & Dubinsky, A. J. (1994). Transformational leadership theory: Using levels of analysis to determine boundary conditions. *Personnel Psychology, 47*, 787–811.

Yokochi, N. (1989). *Leadership styles of Japanese business executives and managers: Transformational and transactional.* Unpublished doctoral dissertation, United States International University, San Diego, CA.

Yukl, G. (2010). *Leadership in organizations* (7th ed). Upper Saddle River, NJ: Prentice Hall.

CHAPTER 7

Issues in Leadership

Brent J. Goertzen

Leadership is a potent combination of strategy and character. If you must be without one, be without the strategy.

H. Norman Schwarzkopf (from *http://thinkexist.com*)

INTRODUCTION

The Global Strategy Institute of the Center for Strategic International Studies, a prestigious think tank in Washington, DC, has identified seven key challenges that policy makers, business figures, and other leaders must address by the year 2025 (Center for Strategic International Studies, 2010). The challenges, known as "Seven Revolutions," include (1) population, (2) resource management, (3) technology, (4) information, (5) economic integration, (6) conflict, and (7) governance. For example, in the area of resource management, the Institute reports that scarcity of resources, such as food and water, will increase as a result of the pressures of a growing population. Furthermore, the current reliance on hydrocarbon-based energy sources will stress the ability to cope with increasing demands. New energy sources are needed to manage these ever-increasing demands. In a rapidly growing, interdependent world, these seven "revolutions" present both major challenges and significant opportunities for people to work together as members of the global human race.

The ability to work together is dictated, in part, by the ability to understand similarities and differences on both moral and cultural grounds. This chapter presents an overview of several important trends and ideas regarding ethics and culture as they pertain to leadership. The section regarding ethics and leadership briefly describes ethical theory, draws connections to moral values from contemporary leadership theories, and explains some emerging research in ethical leadership. The culture and leadership section describes cultural dimensions and a major research project that integrates cultural dimensions and effective leadership traits and behaviors.

ETHICS AND LEADERSHIP

There has been increasing coverage in the popular press and news media of fallen leaders. In every realm of life, from business to politics, from education to medicine, from the military to religion, there are fallen leaders tarnished by moral scandals (Johnson, 2009). It seems that everywhere are found leaders who do not live up to society's moral expectations. Such examples as the bankruptcy of Enron, the physical and psychological abuse of detainees in the Abu Ghraib prison, and the Ponzi scheme orchestrated by Bernie Madoff all serve as wretched reminders of unethical leadership. However, these examples also cause one to assert that ethics is at the heart of leadership (Ciulla, 1998).

This section addresses several important issues regarding the understanding of ethics in leadership. First described are factors that contribute to moral failings. Then, moral theory is examined, and its intersection with several contemporary leadership theories is described. Finally, the landscape of current research regarding ethical leadership is reviewed.

Leadership Points to Ponder

What lies behind us and what lies before us are tiny matters compared to what lies within us.

Ralph Waldo Emerson (from *http://thinkexist.com*)

Toxic Triangle of Unethical Leadership

Padilla, Hogan, and Kaiser (2007) postulated a model of three critical elements (destructive leaders, susceptible followers, and conducive environments) that together set the stage for leadership that is unethical in both motives and actions. This destructive form of leadership has a selfish orientation, involves control and coercion, and yields tremendously destructive outcomes that compromise the quality of life for constituents.

Destructive leaders

The model asserts that destructive leaders are characterized by five criteria: (1) charisma, (2) personalized use of power, (3) narcissism, (4) negative life themes, and (5) an ideology of hate. Such leaders use their charisma and self-presentation skills to build support for themselves and enhance their personal power. Leaders with personalized power need to use authority "in an impetuously aggressive manner for self-aggrandizing purpose, to the detriment of their subordinates and organizations" (House & Aditya, 1997, p. 414). Narcissism reinforces the personalized use of power, because leaders suffering from narcissistic tendencies offer grandiose dreams for success and power but ignore key external environmental factors or tests of judgment. Negative life themes experienced by exploitive adults may include parental discord, low socioeconomic status, parental criminality, maternal or paternal psychiatric disorder, and child abuse (Hare

1993). Furthermore, images of hate are contained in the rhetoric, vision, and worldview of destructive leaders (Padilla et al., 2007). These images revolve around the notions of "vanquishing rivals" and "destroying despised enemies." Each of these qualities alone may not cause a leader to be destructive; however, these characteristics are theorized to interact to form a potentially dangerous leader.

Leadership Points to Ponder

Every man must decide whether he will walk in the light of creative altruism or in the darkness of destructive selfishness.

Martin Luther King, Jr. (from *http://thinkexist.com*)

Susceptible followers

Scholars suggest that some followers need safety, security, group members, and predictability in an uncertain environment and therefore are unwilling or unable to resist a domineering or abusive leader (Kellerman, 2004). There are two general types of susceptible followers of destructive leaders: conformers and colluders (Padilla et al., 2007). Conformers passively stand by while the leader assumes power. Their unmet basic needs, negative self-esteem, and immaturity cause them to be vulnerable to leaders motivated by power. Colluders, however, support and perhaps even actively participate alongside the destructive leader. Motivated by ambition for status, colluders engage in exploitive behavior because of unsocialized values, such as greed and selfishness, or they may find their beliefs consistent with those of the destructive leader.

Conducive environments

A conducive environment, the third component of the toxic triangle, comprises four critical aspects: (1) instability, (2) perceived threat, (3) cultural values, and (4) the absence of checks and balances. Leaders assuming control during periods of instability are typically granted more authority to make unilateral decisions to act quickly (Vroom & Jago, 1974). Objective threats are not necessary to help shape a conducive environment; all that is needed is the perception of a threat. Destructive leaders can exploit perceived threats to galvanize power and motivate followers. Some cultural values may also help shape the context for the rise of destructive leaders. For instance, cultures that endorse avoidance of uncertainty, collectivism, and high "power distance" between those of high and low status are proposed to foster an environment conducive to destructive leaders (Luthans, Peterson, & Ibrayeva, 1998). Finally, an environment that lacks an appropriate system of checks and balances can create a culture of apathy among followers, which in turn contributes to the centralization of power. Such an environment, "particularly when combined with instability and ineffective institutions, concentrates power in a leader, leading to greater follower dependence and weakening of opposition and dissidence" (Padilla et al., 2007, p. 186).

Leadership Points to Ponder

What type of leadership environment does your workplace have?

Think of ways you can bring your leadership skills to the forefront to create a healthier and more collaborative environment.

Ethics and Effectiveness

Prior chapters in this book have examined various conceptualizations and evaluations of leadership. Most of these perspectives seek to describe and explain two salient questions: What is leadership, and how is it effective? Limited attention has been paid to what constitutes good leadership. Perhaps it goes without saying that leadership can be ethical but not effective, just as it can be effective without being ethical. All too often, "in leadership, one is tempted to put what is effective before what is ethical. We hope for leaders who know when ethics should and shouldn't take priority over effectiveness" (Ciulla, 2003, p. xiii). Distinctions between how people think about ethical and effective leadership help one to understand what Ciulla called "the Hitler problem." Take a moment to answer the question "Was Hitler a good leader?." If we conceptualize leadership only in terms of effectiveness, the answer is yes, because he was

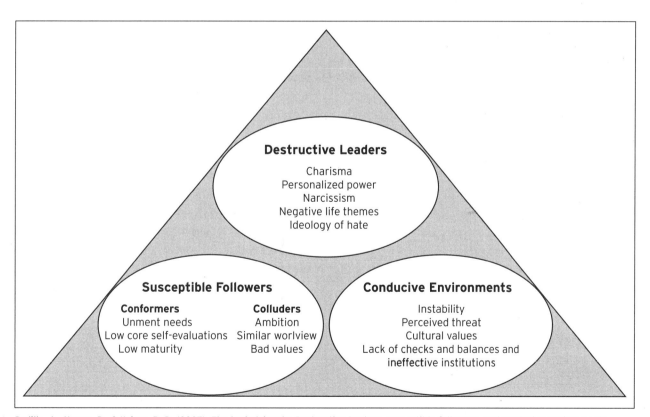

Padilla, A., Hogan, R., & Kaiser, R. B. (2007). The toxic triangle: Destructive leaders, susceptible followers, and conducive environments. *Leadership Quarterly, 18*(30) 180. Reprinted with permission from Pergamon.

Figure 7-1 Toxic Triangle: Domains Relevant to Destructive Leadership.

able to get people together to perform a complicated and difficult task. If we conceptualize leadership in terms of ethics, the answer to that same question is very different because the task was an immoral one and was performed by immoral means. Ciulla asserted that good leadership "depends on the ethics of the means and ethics of the ends of the leader's actions.... Most of us want leaders who do the right thing, the right way, for the right reasons and are personally moral" (Ciulla, 2003, p. xiv).

A Brief Summary of Moral Theory

For the purpose of examining ethics and leadership, we can consider ethical theory that revolves around two general categories: moral action and moral agent. Within the broad category of moral action is ethical theory that focuses on the means and ends of moral action. *Means* refers to the leader's conduct. *Ends* refers to the consequences or outcome of that conduct. Ethical theory that focuses on the moral agent is referred to as virtue (character-based) ethics. **TABLE 7-1** provides an overview of the general categories of ethical theory.

Duty ethic (deontologic theory)

Duty ethic (deontologic theory) dictates that individuals must determine appropriate means to achieve the ends. Deontology is derived from the Greek *deont*, meaning "binding." Deontologic doctrine maintains that the concept of "duty" is independent of the concept of "good" (Beauchamp & Bowie, 1979). This branch of ethics deals with moral obligation, duty, and right action. For example, a contractual relationship is a form of promise keeping, and the "binding" obligation of promises is independent of consequences. Other general duties include the duty to tell the truth and to protect human life (Ciulla, 2003).

Utilitarian theory (greatest good)

It is difficult to consider leadership without evaluating the greatest good for the greatest number of people (Ciulla, 2003). Considered the "principle of greatest

Table 7-1 General Categories of Ethical Theory

Moral Action	Moral Agent
Means Duty ethics (deontology)	Character Virtue ethics
Consequences (ends) Utilitarianism	

happiness," utilitarian doctrine holds that actions are considered right actions to the extent that they promote the greatest happiness (Mill, 1962). According to utilitarian theory, pleasure and freedom from pain are the only desirable ends. Actions are considered right if they maximize pleasure or happiness or minimize pain. Put differently, the right act, or the act that ought to be done, is the act that will maximize happiness; this, then, is the act of greatest utility (Finnis, 1983). The "maximization of good" principle suggests that one ought always to produce the greatest possible value of good for all persons affected. Utilitarian theory measures good as "quantitative units of individual happiness" that are "determined by considering the intensity, the duration, the certainty, or uncertainty, the nearness or remoteness, the fecundity, the purity, and the extent of any proposed action or event" (Beauchamp & Bowie, 1979, p. 5). Accordingly, the multiplication of happiness is considered the greatest virtue (Mill, 1962).

Character (ethic of virtue)

Perhaps the first individuals to explicitly address the ethics of virtue were the ancient Greek philosophers Sophocles, Plato, and Aristotle. Aristotle defined virtue as a trait of character manifested in habitual action. Aristotle believed that virtues, such as courage, were important because the virtuous person would fare better in life. Referring to Aristotle's concept of virtue, Whetstone identified three conditions for an act to be considered virtuous:

1. The virtuous person *does the act knowingly*, aware of the pertinent facts and the practical wisdom needed to apply the act so as to fit its appropriate purpose;

2. The motive for choosing the act must be simply *because it is virtuous*, not for personal advantage or other non-ideal motives; and

3. The act must be as a result of a *steady state of character* disposition, not a one-off or impulsive act, but irrespective of particular times and persons.

A virtuous act is thus a *rational act* based on a *wise, purposeful assessment* of the factual situation, chosen for a *pure motive*, and consistent with a *steady disposition* of the actor's character (*emphasis added*; Whetstone, 2001, p. 104).

It seems obvious that virtues may be thought of as differing from person to person. Rachels (1999) recognized that traits of character are needed to occupy different roles in different contexts of societies; thus, it seems reasonable to argue that virtues are different. However, this notion may be countered by the idea that "there are some virtues that will be needed by all people in all times" (p. 186). An argument can be made that everyone, in every time, needs such virtues as courage, generosity, honesty, and loyalty. Rachels identified the rationale for these particular four virtues as follows:

1. Everyone needs courage because no one is so safe that danger may not sometimes arise.

2. In every society there will be property to be managed and decisions to be made about who gets what, and in every society there will be some people who are worse off than others, so generosity is always to be prized.

3. Honesty in speech is always a virtue because no society can exist without communication among its members.

4. Everyone needs friends, and to have friends one must be a friend, so everyone needs loyalty. (Rachels, 1999, p. 186–187)

Leadership Points to Ponder

The supreme quality for leadership is unquestionably integrity. Without it, no real success is possible no matter whether it is on a section gang, a football field, in an army or in an office.

Dwight David Eisenhower (from *http://thinkexist.com*)

Leadership Theories and Moral Requirements of Leadership

Several of the leadership perspectives described in previous chapters of this book have either explicitly or implicitly integrated moral values into their frameworks. This section delineates these values per several of these contemporary leadership theories.

Burns's transforming leadership theory

Burns's perspective of transforming leadership revolutionized the way scholars and practitioners thought of leadership, in large part because it brought ethics to the forefront of the discussion of what leadership is and how it should be carried out. Burns explicitly involves ethical requirements in his understanding of leadership. Burns defined leadership as when "one or more persons engage with others in such a way that leaders and followers raise one another to higher levels of motivation and morality" (Burns, 1979, p. 20). Clearly, this perspective places in high regard followers' needs, values, and morals. Therefore, it is inherently grounded in moral foundations (Bass & Steidlmeier, 1999). The moral principles stressed by Burns include end values, such as liberty, justice, and equality.

Bass and Steidlmeier (1999) differentiated "pseudo-transformational leaders" from "authentic transformational leaders." Pseudotransformational leaders are described as deceptive and manipulative. Authentic transformational leaders are considered moral because they refrain from coercion, but rather focus on persuading others based on the merits of issues. Furthermore, leadership requires altruistic motivation in that it emphasizes followers' needs. Bass (1998) noted that:

Leaders are authentically transformational when they increase awareness of what is right, good, important, and beautiful, when they help elevate followers' needs for achievement and self-actualization, when they foster in followers higher moral maturity, and when they move followers to go beyond their self-interests for the good of their group, organization, or society. (p. 171)

Rost's postindustrial paradigm

Rost (1993) proposed the following highly promising definition of leadership: "an influence relationship among leaders and followers who intend real changes that reflect their mutual purposes" (p. 102). This postindustrial paradigm of leadership is based on four components: (1) the relationship is based on influence, (2) leaders and followers are people in this relationship, (3) leaders and followers intend real changes, and (4) leaders and followers develop mutual purposes. Disappointingly, he asserted that there were no moral requirements within this framework because, as he considered it, moral requirements are "too limiting, and thus unacceptable" (p. 124). For Rost, "the changes that leaders and followers intend can fall along a continuum of morality" (p. 124).

Leadership Points to Ponder

Character cannot be developed in ease and quiet. Only through experience of trial and suffering can the soul be strengthened, vision cleared, ambition inspired, and success achieved.

Helen Keller (from *http://thinkexist.com*)

Nonetheless, although Rost attempts to exclude moral requirements from his perspective of leadership, his perspective is inherently laden with moral values. For example, leadership that requires leaders and followers to refrain from using coercive pressure to influence others essentially prohibits the abuse of power and both acknowledges and respects the autonomy and "free will" of participants to engage (or not to engage) in the leadership process. Additionally, according to Rost, leaders and followers are obligated to develop mutual aims and purposes. Another moral value is seen undergirding this component of leadership because it prohibits leaders from imposing self-interest. Leadership must include altruistic motivations of both leaders and followers to develop shared purposes for change.

Greenleaf's servant leadership

Greenleaf developed the concept of leader as servant in the 1970s. Servant leadership emphasizes service to others and to community and proposes that those being led will "become healthier, wiser, freer, more autonomous [and] more likely themselves to become servants" (Greenleaf, 1977, p. 13). Within this paradigm of leadership, leaders emerge by demonstrating care for others. Servant leaders are exceedingly attentive to the concerns of followers, empathize with them, and help them to grow to higher levels of maturity.

In addition to possessing an extraordinary concern for the needs of others, servant leaders put their calling into action by displaying a deep commitment to social responsibility. Servant leaders are attuned to the unequal power distribution that exists between stakeholders, and they seek to correct inequities and remove social injustices (Graham, 1991). This type of leader influences others not with formal authority, but through personal credibility and trust earned by service to others and the building of community.

Leadership Points to Ponder

In Greenleaf's writings, he mentions that the early Roman leadership style was to be first among equals. How could this style of leadership be used in today's world?

Relevant Qualities of Ethical Leaders
Courage

Ancient philosophers originally defined moral courage as limiting one's fear of the loss of ethical integrity and authenticity (Putman, 1997). Courage is the willingness to persevere in the face of challenging situations and substantial consequences. Courage is essentially the limiting of fears that hold one back in difficult situations, despite following reason's lead.

For Aristotle, courage resides in the realm of confidence and fear. The excess of confidence is rashness, or foolhardiness, and its deficiency is cowardice; courage, therefore, is the median point between these two extremes. The individual who is involved in an event of great danger and meets the situation with proper spirit is more courageous than the individual who behaves similarly under encouraging circumstances. Courage is the capacity to know and understand one's strengths and limitations within a reasonable probability of success for a given situation.

There is a difference between physical and moral courage. Physical courage refers to remaining steadfast in situations involving physical or bodily harm. Moral courage is defined as "the quality of mind and spirit that enables one to face up to ethical dilemmas and moral wrongdoings firmly and confidently, without flinching or retreating" (Kidder & Bracy, 2001, p. 5). Moral courage is connected with social disapproval (Martin, 1986; Walton, 1986). Therefore, individuals motivated by moral courage attempt to maintain moral integrity while at the same time overcoming the fear of rejection by friends or colleagues. Examples of moral courage often occur in the workplace. The whistle-blower attempting to draw attention to injustices in the workplace may face ostracism by coworkers and colleagues (Putman, 1997). As a result, an individual primarily motivated by moral courage may not substantially consider the social consequences of the situation and may therefore hinder the quality of relations with coworkers.

Leadership Points to Ponder

Part of every decision about moral courage, then, involves some form of that starkly famous military question: Is this the hill you want to die on? Is this issue in fact the big one? If you must hazard all—house, family, children, job, career, financial future—is this the mast on which to nail your colors?

Rushworth Kidder (2006, p. 136)

Reflect on the quotation by Rushworth Kidder and consider: On what "mast" would you be willing to "nail your colors"?

Trustworthiness

Trustworthiness is the result of truthful and genuine social interactions. Aristotle believed that a trustworthy individual is sincere, communicates truthful information, and lives life in a consistent manner. However, the primary foundation for trustworthiness remains honest communication. The trustworthy individual refrains from deceit because "deceptive truths" and lies seem to be morally indistinguishable (Rachels, 2003). Trust does not imply that one ought to trust everyone; rather, trust is built on experience and judgment from an expectation of trustful relationships. The trustworthy individual strives to remain truthful in social interactions.

The development of trustworthiness depends largely on the history of one's interpersonal relationships. Based on this consideration, "trust thickens or thins as a function of the cumulative history of interaction between interdependent parties" (Kramer, 1996, p. 218). Trust is believed to play an important role in the development of quality relationships (Butler, 1991). Butler defined eleven behaviors associated with interpersonal trust:

1. Availability
2. Competence
3. Consistency
4. Discreetness
5. Fairness
6. Integrity
7. Loyalty
8. Openness
9. Promise fulfillment
10. Receptivity
11. Overall trust

People's desire for trust is reflected in their behavior. As a result, people who are strongly motivated by trustworthiness likely display behaviors aimed at influencing others' perceptions of trustworthiness in them.

Loyalty

Loyalty refers to the sense that one can be counted on by others. Loyalty may be directed toward different individuals, groups, or entities, such as family, coworkers, supervisors or subordinates, work groups, organizations, or even nations. Solomon (1992) indicated that loyalty is a form of integrity and conceiving oneself as part of a larger group organization or community. Possible reciprocal effects can be gained from the development of loyalty. For example, psychological benefits may accrue that shape and enhance self-esteem (Rachels, 2003).

Fairness

Fairness includes the notions of equality and impartiality. An individual with a developed sense of fairness is able to consider the interests of all parties without the influence of favoritism. Fairness can be thought of as the equality in the distribution of outcomes of the ethical decision (Schminke, Ambrose, & Noel, 1997). The basic rule of fairness holds that differentiated treatment of individuals should not be based on arbitrary characteristics (Cavanagh, Moberg, & Velasquez, 1981). In essence, the rules of fairness serve to strike a balance between conflicting interests. Ethical leaders are able to apply these rules of fairness as they encounter ethical dilemmas.

Justice

Justice signifies equality, to adjust something by making it equal to some standard. Justice here refers to the motivating disposition that leads one to adhere to moral integrity with respect to policies, rules, or laws within a community. A system of laws provides an illustration of procedural justice. For example, rather than debate the fairness of each individual punishment, the debate shifts to the best criteria for a just procedure. Procedural justice refers to decisions made in congruence with appropriate rules, regulations, or laws that might apply to given circumstances.

Care

Care is an attitude of affection and involves an emotional bond that creates a sense of belonging and attachment to other human beings (Solomon, 1992). Concepts related to caring include love and generosity. Kidder (1994) asserted that individuals ought to value love. Respondents in Kidder's investigation indicated that the world needs love more than anything else. Rachels (2003) makes the case that generosity is an essential virtue across time and cultures. It is likely that generosity is a function, or an outcome, of caring, which would direct the behaviors of altruism and benevolence to particular individuals.

Leadership Points to Ponder

There is more hunger for love and appreciation in this world than for bread.

Mother Teresa (from *http://thinkexist.com*)

Gilligan (1977) was the first researcher to investigate the notion of an ethic of care. A common thread throughout the ethic of care is ensuring that no one gets hurt and refraining from doing harm to others. Moral judgment based on caring "stresses the necessity to be responsible to relationships, to be sensitive to others' needs, and to avoid causing pain" (Kuk, 1990). Furthermore, the ethic of care nurtures growth and development in others (Puka, 1988).

Ciulla (2009) asserted that caring is not limited to the realm of emotions but may also inform one's sense of duty. "'Being there' means the leader is 'on the job' and paying attention. A leader's presence can give followers confidence in the leader and this confidence can be a source of comfort" (p. 4).

Leadership Points to Ponder

Labour to keep alive . . . that little spark of celestial fire called conscience.

George Washington
(from *http://www.quotationspage.com*)

Responsibility

Individuals take on different degrees of responsibility. For instance, an individual may demonstrate commitment to a work unit, department, or organization by getting involved in the political life of the organization. Other individuals may demonstrate local, community, state and regional, national, or global responsibility by becoming involved in the civic life of these various arenas.

Responsibility cannot exist without the notion of accountability. Josephson (2002) explained this connection well by asserting that an individual with a strong moral character demonstrates responsibility because they prudently evaluate and accept the potential consequences of their actions. Additionally, responsible moral agents do not accept credit for the work of others and do not shift blame for their failures to others.

Leadership Points to Ponder

Do you take responsibility for problems that arise in the workplace or at home? Leaders who take responsibility gain the trust of those who follow them.

Research in Ethics and Leadership

Although there has been a substantial amount of theory developed drawing the connections between ethics and leadership, there has yet to be much empirical research examining the nature and consequences of ethical leadership (Ciulla, 1998). This section describes some of these studies.

One such study examined the contrast between an ethic of care and an ethic of justice as these orientations pertain to leadership (Simola, Barling, & Turner, 2010). The study treated the ethics of care and justice as moral orientations, and hence character traits. They reported that leaders who were disposed to an ethic of justice were more likely to demonstrate transactional leader behaviors. However, leaders who were motivated by an ethic of care were more likely to be transformational.

Perhaps some of the most promising systematic treatment of the subject of ethical leadership is the research being conducted by Brown and Trevino and colleagues. They have looked at ethical leadership from a descriptive ethics position rather than a normative perspective. A normative perspective specifies how leaders ought to behave, whereas a descriptive perspective describes how they do behave.

Trevino, Brown, and Hartman (2003) conducted in-depth interviews with CEOs and ethics compliance officers of medium to large American companies. They reported that ethical leaders demonstrate five general categories of behavior: (1) exhibiting a people orientation and concern for others, (2) displaying visible ethical actions and traits, (3) establishing and maintaining ethical standards and accountability, (4) showing a broad ethical awareness, and (5) adhering to sound decision-making processes.

Research that followed this line of inquiry investigated how ethical leadership was related to organizational outcomes (Brown, Trevino, & Harrison, 2005). They defined ethical leadership as "the demonstration of normatively appropriate conduct through personal actions and interpersonal relationships, and the promotion of such conduct to followers through two-way communication, reinforcement, and decision-making" (p. 120). They reported that leaders engaged in ethical leadership were more likely to display consideration behaviors and be more fair and honest than other leaders. Employees reported having greater satisfaction with and more trust in the leader. Furthermore, employees perceived ethical leaders as being more effective and were more willing to exert extra effort for them.

Strengths

Ethical leadership offers a number of critical strengths. First and foremost, it is timely (Northouse, 2010). In the current era, people expect and demand their leaders to possess higher levels of moral responsibility than ever before. In today's information society, there is tremendous access to the personal lives of leaders whereby "every wart and wrinkle of a person's life is public.... The more defective our leaders are, the greater our longing to have more highly ethical leaders" (Ciulla, 1998, p. 3).

Another important strength of this domain of leadership is that it challenges the thinking about what constitutes good leadership. Very few leadership perspectives described in the preceding chapters explicitly emphasize the importance of moral values; most seek only to explain what constitutes effective leadership. When one thinks of leadership in terms of ethics, it may radically alter the understanding of the content, process, and outcomes of leadership.

Weaknesses and Limitations

Ethical leadership as a theory is not without weaknesses. First and foremost, there is still very limited research in this area. There are a number of published studies in business ethics research; however, very little has integrated ethics and leadership (Northouse, 2010). Ciulla noted, "it's remarkable that there has been little in the way of sustained and systematic treatment of the subject [of ethics and leadership] by scholars" (Ciulla, 1998, p. 3). More recently, she reported that there has been little progress in the state of leadership ethics because "the literature in this area is still quite small" (Ciulla, 2005, p. 323).

A related weakness is that the literature is heavily influenced by the writing of just a few scholars. Northouse (2010) noted that this area of leadership is largely based on "personal opinions about the nature of leadership ethics and their view of the world" (p. 394) and therefore lacks the empirical support that accompanies other perspectives of leadership.

CULTURE AND LEADERSHIP

Sensitivity to cultural issues is of paramount importance in today's global markets. However, many of the key leadership concepts and theories emerged from research conducted primarily in the United States. "In a global perspective, U.S. management theories contain a number of idiosyncrasies not necessarily shared by management elsewhere. Three such idiosyncrasies are mentioned: A stress on market processes, a stress on the individual and a focus on managers rather than workers" (Hofstede, 1993, p. 81). As such, it is reasonable to assume that different cultural groups may vary in their conceptions of important characteristics of leaders and what constitutes effective leadership.

Despite the intuitive expectation that notions of leadership would vary across cultures, some scholars assert that there are commonalities. Bass (1997) argued that transformational leadership transcends national and cultural bounds because it is related to many positive organizational outcomes. Bass's proposition has been supported by research conducted in diverse countries such as the United States, India, Spain, Japan, China, New Zealand, and the Netherlands. Other studies also have reported consistencies in the profiles of effective leadership across cultures (e.g., Den Hartog, House, Hanges, Ruiz-Quintanilla, & Dorfman, 1999).

The GLOBE Project

The Global Leadership and Organizational Behavior Effectiveness (GLOBE) project is a cross-cultural study examining leadership in more than 60 countries representing all major regions of the world (House et al., 2004). It is an ongoing project originally launched in 1991 by lead scholar Robert House that has included more than 150 researchers in different countries. This comprehensive research project explores cultural values and practices and identifies their impact on leadership behaviors and attributes. Several of the driving research questions are as follows:

- Are there leader behaviors and attributes and organizational practices that are universally accepted and effective across cultures?

- Are there leader behaviors and attributes and organizational practices that are accepted and effective in only some cultures?

- How do attributes of societal and organizational cultures affect the kinds of leader behaviors and organizational practices that are accepted and effective? (House & Javidan, 2004, p. 10)

Dimensions of culture

The GLOBE project defines culture as "shared motives, values, beliefs, identities, and interpretations or meanings of significant events that result from common experiences of members of collectives that are transmitted across generations" (House et al., 2004, p. 15). The study identified nine dimensions of culture.

1. Power distance
2. Uncertainty avoidance
3. Humane orientation
4. Institutional collectivism
5. In-group collectivism
6. Assertiveness
7. Gender egalitarianism
8. Future orientation
9. Performance orientation

Participants in the study respond to questions about current practices in their organizations and what "should be" to evaluate values of the organization. A similar process is conducted regarding societal practices and values.

Power distance: Power distance refers to the emphasis that a community places on differences in power and status privileges. Essentially, this dimension deals with human equality and reflects the degree to which a culture expects that power should be shared equally. In addition to power, equality may also reflect differences in other areas, such as prestige, wealth, or status.

Uncertainty avoidance: Uncertainty avoidance regards the extent to which individuals feel threatened or anxious in ambiguous situations. Collectives that seek to avoid uncertainty encourage individuals to search for consistency and structure. Cultures reporting high levels of this dimension emphasize laws, rules, or other policies that promote predictable and orderly behavior.

Humane orientation: Humane orientation reflects how individuals within a culture treat one another. Cultures demonstrating high levels of humane organization emphasize being fair, kind, altruistic, and compassionate to one another. Additionally, individuals in this type of culture feel responsible for helping and promoting the well-being of others.

Institutional collectivism: Institutional collectivism refers to the degree to which a culture encourages collective action. Individuals in cultures reporting high levels of this dimension tend to sacrifice personal goals and desires to help others.

In-group collectivism: In-group collectivism refers to the degree to which individuals express pride in and loyalty to their organizations. This dimension is more focused on organizations and families than institutional collectivism, which focuses on the societal level.

Assertiveness: Assertiveness is the degree to which individuals in a culture are aggressive, dominant, or tough in social situations. Cultures reporting high levels of assertiveness tend to value competition and direct and unambiguous communication. Additionally, individuals in these cultures are encouraged to express thoughts and feelings.

Gender egalitarianism: Gender egalitarianism refers to the degree to which a culture seeks to minimize gender role differences. Cultures high on gender egalitarianism tend to have more women in positions of authority, afford women a greater role in community decision making, and have a higher percentage of women working in the labor force.

Future orientation: Future orientation relates to the subjective experience of time. Cultures that have a high level of future orientation value planning and delaying gratification. This cultural orientation emphasizes the capabilities and willingness of long-term planning. Such cultures may delay gratification to develop strategies to meet enduring aspirations.

Performance orientation: Performance orientation reflects the degree to which a community or collective fosters and rewards high standards of excellence and improvement. Cultures that score high on this dimension tend to believe that anyone can succeed if he or she works hard enough; value performance more than status; and place a premium on initiative, assertiveness, and competiveness.

Clusters of cultures and their characteristics

The GLOBE project has identified a set of 10 regional clusters. These clusters aided in the analysis and understanding of the similarities and differences between societies. Regional clusters were determined using prior research (Ronen & Shenkar, 1985) that used such factors as religion, language, geography, ethnicity, and work-related values. A list of clusters and the countries in each cluster are identified.

1. **Anglo**: Canada, the United States, Australia, Ireland, England, South Africa (white sample), New Zealand

2. **Germanic Europe**: Austria, the Netherlands, Switzerland, Germany

3. **Latin Europe**: Israel, Italy, Switzerland (French speaking), Spain, Portugal, France

4. **Sub-Saharan Africa**: Zimbabwe, Namibia, Zambia, Nigeria, South Africa (black sample)

5. **Eastern Europe**: Greece, Hungary, Albania, Slovenia, Poland, Russia, Georgia, Kazakhstan

6. **Middle East**: Turkey, Kuwait, Egypt, Morocco, Qatar

7. **Confucian Asia**: Singapore, Hong Kong, Taiwan, China, South Korea, Japan

8. **Southern Asia**: Philippines, Indonesia, Malaysia, India, Thailand, Iran

9. **Latin America**: Ecuador, El Salvador, Colombia, Bolivia, Brazil, Guatemala, Argentina, Costa Rica, Venezuela, Mexico

10. **Nordic Europe**: Denmark, Finland, Sweden

Researchers analyzed data from each of the regions on the nine cultural dimensions. They concluded that there was strong support for the theorized clusters (**TABLE 7-2**).

Anglo: The Anglo cluster reported high performance orientation and low in-group collectivism. This suggests that individuals have a high expectation of excellence and achievement and low attachment to organizations and families compared to other clusters.

Germanic Europe: The Germanic European cluster comprises societies where German is spoken. Participants from these countries reported high levels of assertiveness, future orientation, performance orientation, and uncertainty avoidance and low humane orientation and in-group collectivism compared to other clusters. Germanic countries emphasize aggressive, individualistic behavior that is future oriented. Similar to the Anglo cluster, Germanic Europeans have a low attachment to families and organizations due to the low responses or institutionalized collectivism.

Latin Europe: The countries in this cluster were largely influenced by Roman culture. They reported moderate scores on seven of the cultural dimensions. Latin Europe is distinguished only by weak scores on both humane orientation and institutional collectivism. This suggests that individual autonomy is emphasized and lesser value is placed on collective or societal goals.

Sub-Saharan Africa: Countries in this cluster reported high emphasis on humane orientation. People in sub-Saharan Africa emphasize human interdependence and are deeply sensitive to the needs of others, even at the expense of personal interests.

Eastern Europe: The Eastern Europe cluster largely comprises of countries from the former Soviet bloc. Eastern Europeans reported high in-group collectivism, assertiveness, and gender egalitarianism but low performance orientation, future orientation, and uncertainty avoidance. This means that individuals in this culture tend to treat men and women equally and are disposed toward favoring family and organizational goals more than societal goals. However, Eastern Europeans are less concerned about performance excellence and long-term planning than other culture clusters.

Middle East: The Middle Eastern cluster is largely dominated by Islamic influences. Individuals from the Middle East reported high concern for in-group collectivism but low scores on future orientation, gender egalitarianism, and uncertainty avoidance. This culture has highly differentiated roles for men and women and places great pride and importance in family groups. Additionally, individuals in this culture "believe the future unfolds with the will of Allah and must not be approached using instrumental means" (House et al., 2004, p. 200), which may explain the low concern for both future orientation and uncertainty avoidance.

Table 7-2 Cultural Clusters and Societal Practices

Culture Cluster	High Cultural Practice	Low Cultural Practice
Anglo	Performance orientation	Institutional collectivism
Germanic Europe	Uncertainty avoidance Assertiveness Future orientation Performance orientation	Humane orientation Institutional collectivism In-group collectivism
Latin Europe	None	Humane orientation Institutional collectivism
Sub-Saharan Africa	Humane orientation	None
Eastern Europe	In-group collectivism Assertiveness Gender egalitarianism	Uncertainty avoidance Future orientation Performance orientation
Middle East	In-group collectivism	Uncertainty avoidance Gender egalitarianism Future orientation
Confucian Asia	Institutional collectivism In-group collectivism Performance orientation	None
Southern Asia	Humane orientation In-group collectivism	None
Latin America	In-group collectivism	Uncertainty avoidance Institutional collectivism Future orientation Performance orientation
Nordic Europe	Uncertainty avoidance Institutional collectivism Gender egalitarianism Future orientation	Power distance In-group collectivism Assertiveness

Source: Adapted from House et al. (2004)

Confucian Asia: The Confucian Asian cluster reported average scores on seven of the nine dimensions of culture. This cluster demonstrates high levels of institutional collectivism, in-group collectivism, and performance orientation. People in these countries tend to emphasize community- or societal-level goals above individual aims and desires. Similarly, they are much more devoted to family than other clusters.

Southern Asia: The Southern Asian cluster is characterized by high levels of humane orientation and in-group collectivism, which reflects a deep concern for families and communities.

Latin America: The Latin American cluster scored high on in-group collectivism but low on performance orientation, future orientation, institutional collectivism, and uncertainty avoidance. This suggests that these cultures "take life as it comes" in dealing with unpredictability and performance. Additionally, people in this cluster tend to highly emphasize loyalty and ties to families, much more so than ties to institutional or societal groups.

Nordic Europe: This cluster is similar to the Germanic European cluster. Nordic European participants reported high future orientation, institutional collectivism, gender egalitarianism, and uncertainty avoidance and low assertiveness, in-group collectivism, and power distance. Nordic people place a high value on equality and long-term success. Assertiveness is downplayed. There is a strong affinity for cooperation and societal goals and far less identification with family groups.

Leadership and culture differences

Coordinators for the regional clusters project assumed that the cultures they were studying endorsed implicit leadership theory (Lord & Maher, 1991). This theory asserts that "individuals have implicit beliefs, convictions, and assumptions concerning attributes and behaviors that distinguish leaders from followers, effective leaders from ineffective leaders, and moral leaders from evil leaders" (House et al., 2004, p. 16).

The GLOBE project identified 22 primary leader attributes that were universally perceived as enhancing leadership effectiveness and 8 that were universally perceived as impeding leadership effectiveness. Thirty-five other leader attributes were considered culturally contingent, meaning they enhanced leadership effectiveness in some cultures and impeded it in others. **TABLE 7-3** provides a summary of positive, negative, and culturally contingent characteristics of effective leaders.

Leadership behaviors across cultural dimensions

The GLOBE project identified and examined six global leader behaviors (see **TABLE 7-4**) and found that cultures share some common conceptions of effective and ineffective leadership (Javidan, House, & Dorfman, 2004). Charisma and values-based, team-oriented, and participative leader behaviors were generally perceived as contributing to effective leadership across all cultures.

Table 7-3 GLOBE Universally Positive, Universally Negative, and Culturally Contingent Leadership Attributes

Positive leader attributes	Trustworthy	Just	Honest	Foresight
	Plans ahead	Encouraging	Positive	Dynamic
	Motive arouser	Confidence builder	Motivational	Dependable
	Intelligent	Decisive	Effective bargainer	Win-win problem solver
	Administratively skilled	Communicative	Informed	Coordinator
	Team builder	Excellence oriented		
Negative leader attributes	Loner	Asocial	Noncooperative	Irritable
	Nonexplicit	Egocentric	Ruthless	Dictatorial
Culturally contingent attributes	Anticipatory	Ambitious	Autonomous	Cautious
	Class conscious	Compassionate	Cunning	Domineering
	Elitist	Enthusiastic	Evasive	Formal
	Habitual	Independent	Indirect	Individualistic
	Intragroup competitor	Intragroup conflict avoider	Intuitive	Logical
	Micromanager	Orderly	Procedural	Provocateur
	Risk taker	Ruler	Self-effacing	Self-sacrificial
	Sensitive	Sincere	Status-conscious	Subdued
	Unique	Willful	Worldly	

Source: Adapted from House, Hanges, Javidan, Dorfman, and Gupta (2004).

Table 7-4 GLOBE Dimensions of Leader Behaviors and Attitudes

Charismatic and values-based leadership	Reflects the ability to inspire and motivate and to expect high performance outcomes from others based on firmly held core values
Team-oriented leadership	Emphasizes effective team building and implementation of a common purpose or goal among team members
Participative leadership	Reflects the degree to which managers involve others in making and implementing decisions
Humane-oriented leadership	Reflects supportive and considerate leadership but also includes compassion and generosity
Autonomous leadership	Refers to independent and individualistic leadership attributes
Self-protective leadership	Focuses on ensuring the safety and security of the individual and group through status enhancement and face saving

Source: Adapted from House and Javidan (2004).

Self-protective behaviors were generally perceived as inhibiting effective leadership in most cultures. The GLOBE project also concluded that, as with leader attributes, a number of leader behaviors are culturally contingent. Humane-oriented leader behavior was perceived as neutral to only moderately contributing to effective leadership.

GLOBE identified several significant relationships between leader behaviors and dimensions of culture. For instance, charismatic and values-based leader behaviors were positively related to performance orientation, in-group orientation, and gender egalitarianism but negatively related to power distance (Javidan et al., 2004). Team-oriented behaviors were positively related to uncertainty avoidance and in-group orientation. Participative leader behaviors were positively related to performance orientation, gender egalitarianism, and humane orientation but negatively related to uncertainty avoidance and power distance.

Humane-oriented behaviors were positively related to three dimensions of culture: (1) humane orientation, (2) uncertainty avoidance, and (3) assertiveness. Autonomous leader behaviors were positively related to performance orientation but negatively associated with humane orientation and institutional collectivism. Finally, self-protective leader behaviors were positively linked to both power distance and uncertainty avoidance but negatively correlated to gender egalitarianism. **Table 7-5** summarizes

the findings of the connections between leader behaviors and cultural dimensions.

Leadership behaviors within culture clusters

Anglo: The Anglo cluster perceives charismatic and values-based and team-oriented behaviors as contributing the most to effective leadership. Participative behaviors are similarly perceived in a positive light but not as much as the other two styles. Humane-oriented behaviors facilitate effective leadership, but self-protective behaviors inhibit it. In total, effective Anglo leaders display inspirational and team-oriented leader behaviors that foster involvement and participation. However, effective leaders are not likely to engage in status-conscious or face-saving behaviors, because they are perceived as inhibiting leadership. **Table 7-6** provides a summary of leader behaviors reported by culture cluster relative to other clusters.

Latin America: The Latin American cluster views charismatic and values-based and team-oriented leader behaviors as positively related to effective leadership. Participative and humane-oriented behaviors are also important, although not to the same degree. Both autonomous and self-protective behaviors are viewed in a negative light. Together, this indicates that effective Latin American leaders make use of inspirational, values-based behaviors focused on individual and team involvement.

Table 7-5 Relationship Between Leadership and Cultural Dimensions

Leadership Attribute	Cultural Dimension	
	Positively Related to...	Negatively Related to...
Charismatic and values based	Performance orientation In-group orientation Gender egalitarianism	Power distance
Team oriented	Uncertainty avoidance In-group orientation	None
Participative	Performance orientation Gender egalitarianism Humane orientation	Uncertainty avoidance Power distance
Humane oriented	Humane orientation Uncertainty avoidance Assertiveness	None
Autonomous	Performance orientation	Humane orientation Institutional collectivism
Self-protective	Power distance Uncertainty avoidance	Gender egalitarianism

Source: Adapted from House, Hanges, Javidan, Dorfman, and Gupta (2004).

These leaders are not necessarily willing to demonstrate much individualism but are willing to engage in self-protective behaviors when necessary.

Latin Europe: The Latin European culture cluster views both charismatic and values-based and team-oriented behaviors as most likely to contribute to effective leadership. Participative behaviors are also perceived favorably but not as much as the first two. Humane-oriented behaviors are considered slightly favorable, autonomous behaviors are viewed as slightly negative, and self-protective behaviors are deemed highly negative. In sum, effective Latin European leaders demonstrate charisma and values-based behaviors and also emphasize team and other participative leader behaviors. These leaders do not endorse individualism, nor are they likely to emphasize generosity or compassion.

Germanic Europe: The Germanic European cluster is also characterized by charismatic and values-based and team-oriented behaviors. Participative behaviors are viewed positively but are not as important as the first

two. Although autonomous behaviors are regarded as neutral, self-protective behaviors are deemed very negative. Germanic Europeans perceive effective leadership as based on charisma and participation and reject self-protectiveness.

Nordic Europe: The Nordic European cluster regards charismatic and values-based and team-oriented behaviors as contributing to effective leadership. Likewise, participative behaviors are viewed positively but not as much as the other two. Humane-oriented behaviors are perceived in a slightly positive manner. Autonomous behaviors are considered neutral, but self-protective behaviors are seen as extremely negative. All in all, effective Nordic European leaders engage in inspirational, team-focused behaviors. Compared to other cultures, Nordic European leaders are extremely participative and engaging and not concerned with status or other self-centered attributes.

Eastern Europe: The Eastern European cluster ranked charismatic and values-based and team-oriented

Table 7-6 Relationship Between Culture Clusters and Leader Behavior

Culture Cluster	Leader Behavior	
	High	**Low**
Anglo	Charismatic and values based Participative Humane oriented	Self-protective
Latin America	Charismatic and values based Team oriented Self-protective	Autonomous
Latin Europe	Charismatic and values based	Humane oriented Autonomous
Germanic Europe	Charismatic and values based Participative Autonomous	Team oriented Self-protective
Nordic Europe	Charismatic and values based Participative	Humane oriented Self-protective
Eastern Europe	Autonomous Self-protective	Participative
Middle East	Self-protective	Charismatic and values based Team oriented Participative
Sub-Saharan Africa	Humane oriented	Autonomous
Confucian Asia	Team oriented Humane oriented Self-protective	Participative
Southern Asia	Charismatic and values based Humane oriented Self-protective	Participative

NOTE: High and low based on rankings relative to other clusters, not whether they are perceived as contributing to effective or ineffective leadership.

Source: Adapted from House, Hanges, Javidan, Dorfman, and Gupta (2004)

behaviors as the most likely to contribute to effective leadership. Participative and humane-oriented behaviors were also positively linked to effective leadership but not as much as the first two. Autonomous behaviors are viewed neutrally. These results suggest that the Eastern European cluster desires leaders who are inspirational and team oriented yet still present a strong

personal identity. Effective leaders in this culture do not believe in the value of participation and are willing to use self-protective, face-saving behaviors when necessary.

Middle East: Like other cultures, the Middle Eastern cluster perceives charismatic and values-based and team-oriented leader behaviors as contributing to effective leadership, but not to the same degree as other clusters. Humane-oriented behaviors are regarded positively. Self-protective behaviors neither help nor hinder effective leadership, but this category ranked among the highest relative to other clusters. To summarize, effective leaders in the Middle East engage in visionary leadership that embraces their performance-oriented culture. Furthermore, effective leaders take on attributes that endorse the cluster's familial values. Effective leaders are also concerned with participation and the welfare of others but not to the extent of other culture clusters.

Sub-Saharan Africa: The Sub-Saharan African cluster perceives humane-oriented leader behaviors very favorably and ranked this dimension the highest relative to other clusters. Autonomous behaviors ranked relatively low compared to other clusters. Charismatic and values-based behaviors are viewed as contributing to effective leadership; however, autonomous and self-protective behaviors are seen in a negative light. Similar to other clusters, effective leaders in Sub-Saharan Africa will likely engage in an inspirational and team-focused approach. However, they will be especially noted for demonstrating extremely high care, compassion, and generosity and even sacrificing personal interests for the sake of others.

Confucian Asia: The Confucian Asian cluster perceives charismatic and values-based behaviors as contributing to effective leadership. Humane-oriented behaviors are also looked at favorably, but not as much as the other two. Autonomous behaviors are perceived as neutral, but self-protective behaviors are perceived in a slightly negative light. In summary, effective Confucian Asian leaders integrate an inspirational, values-based style with team effort and the needs of others. However, they also emphasize status and are willing to engage in face-saving behaviors when appropriate.

Southern Asia: The Southern Asian cluster also reported that charismatic and values-based and team-oriented behaviors contribute to effective leadership. Likewise, participative and humane-oriented behaviors also facilitate effective leadership, but not as much as the first two. Autonomous behaviors are considered neutral, but self-protective behaviors are viewed very negatively. In sum, Southern Asia sees effective leadership as inspirational, with high levels of involvement and participation, caused in part by a deep-seated care and concern for others. However, leaders are very willing to use face-saving techniques when necessary.

Strengths

There are a number of important strengths related to the GLOBE project and the understanding of culture and leadership. First and foremost, a major strength of this ambitious project is its sheer magnitude and scope. It integrates perceptions of individuals representing more than 60 countries, which helps shed light on similarities and differences in how effective and ineffective leadership is viewed between cultures. Furthermore, it challenges one to consider perceptions of good and bad leadership in different cultures. Additionally, it expands on Hofstede's (1993) cultural dimensions and adds several key dimensions that elaborate on cultural variability (Northouse, 2010). Integrating the nine dimensions of culture offers a more detailed examination of cultural differences.

Weaknesses and Limitations

The GLOBE project has also been criticized for several reasons. For example, although the findings of the project reveal differences in culture and leadership profiles, they do not offer a unifying theory of leadership. Even though relationships are reported between culture clusters and leadership behaviors, the findings lack a clear set of uniform assumptions and propositions on how culture relates to leadership processes (Northouse, 2010). Additionally, despite the added cultural dimensions in the GLOBE study, several of the facets are criticized for vagueness and lack of clarity.

Furthermore, Graen (2006) sharply criticized the process used to aggregate dimensions and cultural profiles. He asserted that "heterogeneous national cultures cannot be described in a representative manner by samples of 300 managers who represent small homogeneous cultural slivers of nations" (p. 97). There are many other factors that influence cultural perceptions of leadership, such as generational differences and differences between educational, social, and economic classes.

Finally, GLOBE was criticized for its choices in grouping the country clusters. For instance, Graen (2006) argued that it is debatable what such countries as China and Japan have in common. He asserted that there are tremendous differences in the business cultures of those two countries and among other countries within clusters.

SUMMARY

Ethics is emerging as a critical component of leadership. This has become especially important with the increased attention to and notoriety of fallen leaders (e.g., Bernie Madoff's Ponzi scheme, the Abu Ghraib prison scandal). Padilla et al. (2007) developed a model of critical elements that set the stage for unethical leadership. They describe the relevance of destructive leaders, acting in concert with susceptible followers and conducive environments that interact in complex ways and foster extremely destructive outcomes.

Ciulla (2003) noted that all too often leadership scholars conceptualize good leadership in terms of its effectiveness rather than the degree to which it is ethical. Effective leadership is not necessarily ethical. When integrating an ethical perspective of leadership, one must be concerned about not only the moral action (the means and ends) of leadership, but also the leader as a moral agent (moral character).

Contemporary leadership theory has begun to integrate aspects of moral values. For example, Burns's (1979) perspective of transforming leadership asserts that leadership elevates both leaders and followers to higher levels of motivation and morality by focusing on end values, such as justice, liberty, and equality. Additionally, Greenleaf's servant leadership model strongly emphasizes altruism in the form of service to others in order that they may become "healthier, wiser, freer, more autonomous and more likely to themselves to become servant leaders" (Greenleaf, 1977, p. 13).

There is emerging yet limited research that describes the qualities of ethical leadership. Trevino et al. (2003) reported that ethical leaders tend to display five general categories of behavior: (1) exhibiting a people orientation and concern for others, (2) displaying visible ethical actions and traits, (3) establishing and maintaining ethical standards and accountability, (4) showing a broad ethical awareness, and (5) adhering to sound decision-making processes.

Subsequent research defined ethical leadership as "the demonstration of normatively appropriate conduct through personal actions and interpersonal relationships, and the promotion of such conduct to followers through two-way communication, reinforcement, and decision-making" (Brown et al., 2005, p. 120). Ethical leadership was related to employee satisfaction and trust in leaders and employees' willingness to exert extra effort for the leader.

The GLOBE project is ambitious research that bridges the domains of culture and leadership. The study identified 9 dimensions of culture and 10 cultural regions across the world. The project identified a number of positive attributes related to effective leadership that are common regardless of cultural differences, such as trustworthy, just, honest, foresight, and encouraging. Attributes generally perceived as negative across cultures include loner, noncooperative, irritable, dictatorial, and egocentric.

Beyond examining traits of effective and ineffective leaders, the GLOBE project also examined similarities and differences regarding leader behaviors. The project identified and defined six dimensions of leader behaviors: (1) charismatic and values based, (2) team oriented, (3) participative, (4) humane oriented, (5) autonomous, and (6) self-protective. In general, charismatic and values-based, team-oriented, and participative behaviors were generally perceived as contributing to effective leadership across cultures. Conversely, self-protective behaviors were typically perceived as inhibiting effective leadership.

Wrap-Up

ACTIVITY

Are You an Ethical Leader?

This activity is intended to challenge you to reflect on your own qualities of being an ethical leader. Answer the following reflection questions based on your current ability for each of the seven qualities of ethical leaders: (1) courage, (2) trustworthiness, (3) loyalty, (4) fairness, (5) justice, (6) care, and (7) responsibility.

1. Which of these capacities have you already developed well? Explain.

2. Which of these capacities do you still need to develop further? Explain.

3. Specify what you can do to further develop these capacities during the next 2 weeks.

Culture and Leadership

Use TABLE 7-5 to identify and create the following

1. Analyze your department's decision-making practices to identify whether leadership decisions typically reflect these six GLOBE dimensions of leader behaviors.

2. After you have gained a thorough understanding of local leadership decision-making practices, create a training exercise for your leadership team to reflect the GLOBE dimensions of leader behaviors.

3. Once you have gained a thorough understanding of local leadership decision-making practices, propose changes to reflect the GLOBE dimensions of leader behaviors.

REFERENCES

Bass, B. M. (1997). Does the transactional-transformational paradigm transcend organizational and national boundaries? *American Psychologist, 52*(2), 130–139.

Bass, B. M. (1998). The ethics of transformational leadership. In J. B. Ciulla (Ed.), *Ethics: The heart of leadership* (pp. 169–192). Westport, CT: Praeger.

Bass, B. M., & Steidlmeier, P. (1999). Ethics, character and authentic transformational leadership behavior. *Leadership Quarterly, 10*(2), 181–217.

Beauchamp, T. L., & Bowie, N. E. (1979). *Ethical theory and business.* Englewood Cliffs, NJ: Prentice-Hall.

Brown, M. E., Trevino, L. K., & Harrison, D. A. (2005). Ethical leadership: A social learning perspective for construct development and testing. *Organizational Behavior and Human Decision Processes, 97,* 117–134.

Burns, J. M. (1979). *Leadership.* New York, NY: Perennial.

Butler, J. K. (1991). Toward understanding and measuring conditions of trust: Evolution of a conditions of trust inventory. *Journal of Management, 17,* 643–663.

Cavanagh, G. F., Moberg, D. J. & Velasquez, M. (1981). The ethics of organizational politics. *Academy of Management Review, 6*(3), 363–374.

Center for Strategic International Studies. (2010). *Seven revolutions: Part of the: Global Strategy Institute.* Retrieved from http://csis.org/program/seven-revolutions

Ciulla, J. B. (1998). *Ethics, the heart of leadership.* Westport, CT: Praeger.

Ciulla, J. B. (2003). *The ethics of leadership.* Belmont, CA: Thompson Wadsworth.

Ciulla, J. B. (2004). *Ethics, the heart of leadership* (2nd ed.). Westport, CT: Praeger.

Ciulla, J. B. (2005). The state of leadership ethics and the work that lies before us. *Business Ethics: A European Review, 14*(4), 323–335.

Ciulla, J. B. (2009). Leadership and the ethics of care. *Journal of Business Ethics, 88,* 3–4.

Den Hartog, D. N., House, R. J., Hanges, P. J., Ruiz-Quintanilla, S. A., & Dorfman, P. W. (1999). Cultural specific and cross-culturally generalizable implicit leadership theories: Are attributes of charismatic/transformational leadership universally endorsed? *Leadership Quarterly, 10*(2), 291–256.

Finnis, J. (1983). *Fundamentals of ethics.* Oxford, UK: Clarendon Press.

Gilligan, C. (1977). In a different voice: Women's conception of self and morality. *Harvard Educational Review, 47*(4), 481–517.

Graen, G. B. (2006). In the eye of the beholder: Cross-cultural lesson in leadership from project GLOBE: A response viewed from the Third Culture Bonding (TCB) model of cross-cultural leadership. *Academy of Management Perspectives, 20*(4), 95–101.

Graham, J. W. (1991). Servant leadership in organizations: Inspirational and moral. *Leadership Quarterly, 2*(2), 105–119.

Greenleaf, R. (1977). *Servant leadership.* New York, NY: Paulist Books.

Hare, R. (1993). *Without conscience: The disturbing world of the psychopaths among us.* New York, NY: Simon & Schuster.

Hofstede, G. (1993). Cultural constraints in management theories. *Academy of Management Executive, 7*(1), 81–94.

House, R., & Aditya, R. (1997). The social scientific study of leadership: Quo Vadis? *Journal of Management, 23,* 409–473.

House, R. J., Hanges, P. J., Javidan, M., Dorfman, P. W., & Gupta, V. (2004). *Culture, leadership and organizations: The GLOBE study of 62 societies.* Thousand Oaks, CA: Sage.

House, R. J., & Javidan, M. (2004). Overview of GLOBE. In R. J. House, P. J. Hanges, M. Javidan, P. W. Dorfman, & V. Gupta (Eds.), *Culture, leadership, and organizations: The GLOBE study of 62 societies* (pp. 9–28). Thousand Oaks, CA: Sage.

Javidan, M., House, R. J., & Dorfman, P. W. (2004). A nontechnical summary of GLOBE findings. In R. J. House, P. J. Hanges, M. Javidan, P. W. Dorfman, & V. Gupta (Eds.), *Culture, leadership, and organizations: The GLOBE study of 62 societies* (pp. 29–48). Thousand Oaks, CA: Sage.

Johnson, C. E. (2009). *Meeting the ethical challenges of leadership: Casting light or shadow* (3rd ed.). Thousand Oaks, CA: Sage.

Josephson M. S. (2002). *Making ethical decisions.* Los Angeles, CA: Josephson Institute for Ethics.

Kellerman, B. (2004). *Bad leadership: What it is, how it happens, and why it matters.* Boston, MA: Harvard Business School Press.

Kidder, R. M. (1994). *Shared values for a troubled world: Conversations with men and women of conscience.* San Francisco, CA: Jossey-Bass.

Kidder, R. M., & Bracy, M. (2001). *Moral courage: A white paper.* Camden, ME: Institute for Global Ethics.

Kidder, R. M. (2006). *Moral courage.* New York, NY: William Morrow.

Kramer, R. M. (1996). Divergent realities and convergent disappointments in the hierarchic relation. Trust and the intuitive auditor at work. In R. M. Kramer & T. R. Tyler (Eds.), *Trust in organizations* (pp. 216–245). Newbury Park, CA: Sage.

Kuk, L. (1990). Perspectives on gender differences. In L. Moore (Ed.), *Evolving theoretical perspectives on students. New directions for student services.* San Francisco, CA: Jossey-Bass.

Lord, R. G., & Maher, K. J. (1991). *Leadership and information processing: Linking perceptions and performance.* Boston, MA: Unwin-Hyman.

Luthans, F., Peterson, S. J., & Ibrayeva, E. (1998). The potential for the "dark side" of leadership in post-communist countries. *Journal of World Business, 33,* 185–201.

Martin, M. (1986). *Self-deception and morality.* Lawrence: University Press of Kansas.

Mill, J. S. (1962). *Utilitarianism, On Liberty, Essay on Bentham, together with selected writings of Jeremy Bentham and John Austin* (Mary Warnock, Ed.). New York, NY: Penguin Books.

Northouse, P. (2010). *Leadership: Theory and practice* (5th ed). Thousand Oaks, CA: Sage.

Padilla, A., Hogan, R., & Kaiser, R. B. (2007). The toxic triangle: Destructive leaders, susceptible followers, and conducive environments. *Leadership Quarterly, 18,* 176–194.

Puka, W. (1988). Ethical caring and development: Pros, cons and possibilities. In S. E. Lee (Ed.). *Inquiries into values* pp. (99–113). Journal Lewiston: Mellen Proceedings.

Putman, D. (1997). Psychological courage. *Philosophy, Psychiatry, and Psychology, 4*(1), 1–11.

Rachels, J. (1999). *The elements of moral philosophy.* New York, NY: McGraw-Hill College.

Rachels, J. (2003). *The elements of moral philosophy* (4th ed.). New York, NY: McGraw-Hill College.

Ronen, S., & Shenkar, O. (1985). Clustering countries on attitudinal dimensions: A review and synthesis. *Academy of Management Review, 10*(3), 435–454.

Rost, J. C. (1993). *Leadership for the 21st century.* New York, NY: Praeger.

Schminke, M., Ambrose, M. L., & Noel, T. W. (1997). The effect of ethical frameworks on perceptions of organizational justice. *Academy of Management Journal, 40*(5), 1190–1207.

Simola, S. K., Barling, J., & Turner, N. (2010). Transformational leadership and leader moral orientation: Contrasting an ethic of justice and an ethic of care. *Leadership Quarterly, 21,* 179–188.

Solomon, R. C. (1992). Corporate roles, personal virtues: An Aristotelian approach to business ethics. *Business Ethics Quarterly, 2*(3), 317–340.

Trevino, L. K., Brown, M., & Hartman, L. P. (2003). A qualitative investigation of perceived ethical leadership: Perceptions from inside and outside the executive suite. *Human Relations, 56*(1), 5–37.

Vroom, B., & Jago, A. (1974). Decision making as a social process: Normative and descriptive models of behavior. *Decision Sciences, 5,* 743–769.

Walton, D. (1986). *Courage: A philosophical investigation.* Berkeley: University of California Press.

Whetstone, J. T. (2001). How virtue fits within business ethics. *Journal of Business Ethics, 33,* 101–114.

3

Leadership Application

CHAPTER

8

In the Heat of Battle

David T. Foster III

Yesterday, December 7th, 1941—a date which will live in infamy—the United States of America was suddenly and deliberately attacked by naval and air forces of the Empire of Japan . . . .

Hostilities exist. There is no blinking at the fact that our people, our territory, and our interests are in grave danger.

With confidence in our armed forces, with the unbounding determination of our people, we will gain the inevitable triumph—so help us God . . . .

Excerpts from Franklin D. Roosevelt's address to Congress,
asking for a declaration of war

INTRODUCTION

When one thinks about leadership in the emergency services today, the word "change" may come to mind. Roles are ever-changing. For those who have been in the public safety profession for a long time, the change may be from one sector to another, such as starting a career in fire service or law enforcement and moving into emergency medical services (EMS). The readers have likely seen many changes in their organizations, changes in personnel, policies, and procedures. On a larger scale, constant changes are seen in how EMS is carried out (e.g., the new EMS Scope of Practice, new certification levels, and new cardiopulmonary resuscitation and emergency cardiac care practices). Change may also be reflected in the way leaders plan, train, and respond to their everyday jobs, such as training on National Incident Management System (NIMS) and other call management processes. This chapter compares and contrasts positional leadership theory under the stress of an emergency situation (transactional leadership) with leadership arising from decisions made by rank-and-file members of an emergency

services organization (situational leadership). How one engages with others is essential in the role of a leader. This chapter provides insight into how one can develop a collaborative partnership with others and appropriately change the leadership approach in different situations.

SCENARIO

It is 8:00 PM on a cold, rainy Saturday night. The tones go off for a multivehicle crash on a major thoroughfare in Anytown, USA. Law enforcement personnel arrive at the scene first and begin to address traffic and crowd control. An engine company arrives and begins to assess the scene and set up command. The company officer realizes that additional resources are needed and calls for additional engine companies, rescue teams, and ambulances. The first ambulance arrives and determines that there are 13 patients, 6 of whom are critical. The senior medic calls for 10 additional ambulances. He too establishes command. A law enforcement shift commander has arrived and directs personnel from this sector to set up traffic

125

control lanes, gather information from drivers and occupants who are not seriously injured, and start the investigation. He also establishes command.

The 911 center is now confused about who is actually in charge at the scene. The jurisdiction does not have a common operations frequency for all responders, and they are getting multiple calls from the three different agency commanders for information and requesting additional resources. Each time one command radios a report, 911 has to confirm with the other command that these are not duplicate requests.

The fire department shift chief arrives and assumes Highway A command. He attempts to establish a staging area and separate EMS and law enforcement sectors. This attempt is futile because neither of those agencies has communications with him except by word of mouth or face-to-face. As additional ambulances arrive, they follow the instructions from their command about where to stage and what vehicles and patients to address. This action frustrates the law enforcement and fire commanders, because their plan for controlling the scene is much different from that of the EMS commander.

The scene is total chaos. No one is actually in charge, and the three entities are arguing about who is in charge and who is to do what. This wastes valuable resources that should be devoted to patient care and other potentially life-threatening safety issues. Law enforcement insists that they are in charge because they are enforcing and investigating the accident. They will determine who is at fault and will spend hours performing investigations and writing reports that will be important for insurance companies and legal judgments. Fire insists that they are the ultimate command because they serve the function of protecting lives and property. The operation has to be coordinated to ensure that hazards are addressed and secured. Extrication functions being performed are the responsibility of the fire department in this jurisdiction, and they insist that they have control until extrication operations are completed and the scene is deemed free of hazards. EMS insists that they are in charge, because there are multiple patients, and patient care and transport take priority over traffic control and scene management.

Future chapters will flash back to this and other scenarios to expand on the situation and clarify when, where, or how a particular leadership approach could be used.

Leadership Points to Ponder

Even though worker capacity and motivation are destroyed when leaders choose power over productivity, it appears that bosses would rather be in control than have the organization work well.

Margaret J. Wheatley
(from *http://www.brainyquote.com*)

COMMAND

When people talk in terms of command, most understand it to mean oversight or control of the incident. The term "command and control" is used to describe management of the scene, or incident management. It focuses on tasks, authority, control, actions, and results and has subordinates who must follow orders to resolve the event. In many ways, each commander in the previous scenario is correct in assuming command for their respective agencies. Each responding service has its own functional perspective and protocols for operating at emergency scenes. Clearly, however, there is no coordinated effort here, which suggests that none of the agencies has performed cross-training to address these differences. The scenario is a classic example of the confusion and harm to human life that can occur without adequate training, coordination, and understanding of local protocol.

Historically, the fire service was the first emergency services agency to embrace a command system in response to wildfires. During the 1970s, fire service command evolved through a series of major wildland fires in California. These large-scale incidents revealed weaknesses in coordination and communications. Many issues were identified, from a lack of common terminology and incompatible communications to inconsistent response plans, which hampered the response to and control of these incidents. The research that followed these incidents led to a formal incident command system that was embraced by the fire service and other public safety agencies to manage their incidents.

The one glaring issue that appeared during this era was that many officers took the command-and-control concept to heart and incorporated it into their daily management regime, rather than using it solely to manage emergency situations. Officers were able to embrace this approach easily, because many had been indoctrinated into their professions via the military, where one person is always in charge. Many officers of this era, and even some today, acted like military drill sergeants. Even though the military model is effective at building accountability, it can also be a demeaning approach in the public sector when applied inappropriately. Unlike military personnel, who are committed to following orders and face grave consequences for not doing so, public safety personnel do have a choice. This author has seen many excellent, or potentially excellent, emergency services providers leave the public safety services sector for other professions because of uncompassionate officers who believed they had the right to scream, yell, and disrespect their personnel based on their rank and status. This trend is changing, ever so slowly, as a new generation of public safety personnel enters the professions with a different understanding of how to manage people and incidents. Leadership education today is more than just command and control; it is also focused on relationships, morals, transparency, vision, and compassion.

APPLICABLE LEADERSHIP THEORIES

Leadership theories guide people based on the type of situation encountered. Some theories are descriptive; others are prescriptive. In the multivehicle crash scenario at the start of this chapter, several leadership theories can be applied, which are discussed later in this chapter. An understanding of management and leadership practices could have helped to resolve interagency interactions before such an incident. Planning and training are essential to all responders understanding their roles and actions in multiagency responses, yet sometimes a poor job is done of performing these processes. NIMS was designed to address these issues. Over this author's 35 years of service, he has seen this scenario play out often. Many people have been taught to take control and manage the operation. The operative word here is "manage." Transactional leadership is derived from management models. Situational leadership could also be related to management models because its methodologies are dictated by followers' maturity. This chapter explores the application of these two theories.

Transactional Leadership

The term "transactional leadership" should immediately bring to mind a transaction. With transactions,

something of value is exchanged for something else of value. Transactional leaders do not take into consideration the needs of their subordinates; they look at what services they can gain in exchange for some type of rewards.

Transactional leadership has a limited place in the public safety professions. Looking back at the chapter scenario, each commander needed to control and accomplish their mission at this scene. The reward to responders and leader was accomplishing the mission with no additional dangers, loss of life, injury to others, and so forth. The first goal was to get the injured to the appropriate care facility. Controlling traffic and nonresponders at the scene required a multiagency approach and, although equally important, protecting all responders from harm is paramount in this incident. The agency commanders were operating as separate entities and practicing transactional leadership because they were focused on only their own missions. Ordering or coercing other responders to do something is a characteristic of transactional leadership.

Emergency services commanders can use transactional leadership to direct most emergency operations. Their primary mission is to get followers to carry out their orders. These leaders are positional in nature, meaning they are leaders (managers) by virtue of their rank or position in the department. Unfortunately, some of these officers use this approach in other situations where the approach is unnecessary and possibly counterproductive, such as ordering around their personnel during station duties or other routine daily activities of the department (situations that are better handled by relationship leadership approaches). First, a look at how transactional leaders can use rewards to influence their personnel's actions.

Rewards can be contingent (contingency rewards) on performance. Most departments conduct some form a promotional process where advancement is decided by testing, feedback from administrators, and in some cases peer reviews. The effort put into preparing for this process can result in the reward of earning the next "badge, bar, or stripe." Sometimes promotion has nothing to do with ability, knowledge, or performance. This author has seen a number of technically competent, well-educated firefighters and paramedics passed over for promotion because their style was to criticize and belittle others rather than encourage them to improve and grow in their positions. Yes, they would have made great scene commanders from a technical standpoint, but they did not demonstrate any relationship-based leadership skills. To be successful, officers have to be skilled in relationship building (humanistic approach) and managing (transactional leadership). They need to be concerned with their followers' emotions, ethics, standards, values (morals), short- and long-term goals, motivations, needs, and desires (transformational leadership). Transactional leadership should be considered as a valuable but limited tool. It can serve one well in command-and-control situations, but when dealing with people (direct reports, professional peers, or constituents) and the broader aims of an organization, one is better served by transformational leadership.

Situational Leadership

As the term implies, situational leadership focuses on how leadership is practiced in various situations. The premise of situational leadership is that different situations may require different approaches by the leader to accomplish goals. Contingency and situational leadership theories describe how different aspects of the situation can enhance or neutralize the leaders' ability to influence employee performance or other organizational outcomes.

Each leader has to evaluate multiple factors that can affect their followers' abilities. Hersey and Blanchard (1988) set forth four approaches to leadership that are used based on the level of support and direction required by followers. The four approaches are divided into two categories: supportive (relationship based) and directive (task behavior based). In emergency services agencies, the directive approach is practiced most frequently during an emergency response, during training, or during functions that require giving directions, establishing priorities, making assignments, setting time lines, and providing clear and concise communications in a manner that is usually in one direction (orders down the chain of command). Subordinates receive the orders and carry out the required tasks to accomplish the objective.

However, the supportive approach is also essential to emergency services leaders. This approach requires leaders to seek feedback from followers and truly listen to their input; coach them to help improve their skills; and praise them for successes and good performance. These techniques build followers' self-worth and pride, boost morale and performance, and strengthen unit cohesion. The supportive approach to leadership requires a relationship between leaders and followers, which leaders need to initiate and take responsibility for building. Although this approach takes perhaps more investment of time and effort than transactional leadership, the results can be impressive for both followers and leaders. Also, it underscores the fact that as a leader, people are the number one resource.

Situational favorableness is broadly defined as "the degree to which the situation itself provides the leader with potential power and influence over the group's behavior" (Fiedler, 1967). According to the contingency model, there are three main situational variables (leader–member relations, task structure, and position power), and the combination of these variables determines the level of situational favorableness. "Leader–member relations" refers to the quality of the relationship between leaders and their employees. Good relations are characterized by friendliness, cooperation, and loyalty. Leader–member relations is thought to have the most impact on situational favorableness. "Task structure" is the extent to which goals and tasks are clearly defined. "Position power" is the extent to which the leader has formal authority to evaluate employee performance and administer rewards and punishments. In the multivehicle crash scenario, which situational variables apply?

The prescriptive nature of situational models of leaderships gives some guidance about which type of leader might be better suited for a certain situation. However, there is a problem with this approach: no single person can fit their personality, perspective, and approach to every situation, yet one is expected by the nature of official rank or position to manage all the situations under their command. Officers who are excellent scene managers may be pitiful at leading their crews in nonemergency situations. The relationship-approach leader may be a little too indecisive in emergency situations. Some may excel in both of these situations but lack political savvy. It is critical to remember that no one theoretical approach to leadership works in every situation; the best leaders know how to read each situation and use the appropriate approach to leadership. Knowledge of situational favorableness variables can help a person to understand their own strengths and weaknesses.

Followers' Roles

What role does the follower play in leadership? Without followers, there is no need for a leader, or leadership. Leader–member exchange theory first appeared in 1975, and its goal is to look at the relationship between the leader and follower. Leader–member exchange theory, at its most simplistic, proposes that when followers feel valued, they are happier and more productive and there is less turnover in the organization. Northouse (2007) cites the work of several researchers in summarizing leader–member exchange:

> *Researchers found that high-quality leader-member exchanges produce less employee turnover, more positive performance evaluations, higher frequency of promotions, greater organizational commitment, more desirable work assignments, better job attitudes, more attention and support for the leader, greater participation, and faster career progress over 25 years (Graen & Uhl-Bien, 1995; Liden, Wayne, & Stilwell, 1993). (p. 155)*

The reader can most likely count on one hand the number of officer classes they have sat through where they were told to respect, care for, and support subordinates.

Everyone is a follower, but not everyone is or can be a leader. Even the highest-ranking officers are followers, because they have to follow the guidance and expectations of those who hire, promote, elect, and hold a stake in them. Leaders also are following those they lead. How is this so? Each person has a capacity to influence the dynamics of any group to which they belong. If the followers reject the leader's ideas and directives, then the leader must change tactics, thus following the lead of the followers' actions. The Merriam-Webster Online Dictionary defines followership as (1) following and (2) the capacity or willingness to follow a leader (Followership, n.d.). According to the second definition, to follow one has to have the desire to do so. Holding rank does not make one a leader; however, that person is, by definition, the group's official or appointed leader. Ranking officers and superiors can manage, but people do not have

to follow; they only have to obey orders. Leaders need follower feedback to lead effectively. Without that feedback, the leader may have trouble indentifying their staff's needs and desires, which could guide the leaders to alter their approaches resulting in a better outcome.

To reach one's leadership potential, one must value personnel and cultivate them through a transformational leadership approach. This approach is dynamic, requiring effort and reciprocity on the part of both leaders and followers. The rewards for such effort include not only the significant benefits described by Northouse, but also the readiness and willingness of personnel to make the transition to leaders seamlessly when a situation calls for it. For example, imagine that a team of firefighters working inside a building during a three-alarm blaze encounters a situation that mandates immediate decision-making and leadership by a member of the crew. If the fire chief has not taught his followers to lead, will one of the firefighters be able to make an executive decision that could save the lives of the entire interior crew? EMS personnel all receive technical training on the procedures to follow in emergency situations; however, by developing followers' competencies to the fullest, they can be taught not only how to follow, but also how to lead when needed.

Leadership Points to Ponder

Consider the people you work with in your crew, sector, or district. Can you identify informal leaders in the group—people who do not hold an appointed rank but whom the rest of the personnel trust and follow? The answer is surely a resounding yes.

To build followers, one needs to focus on developing the capacity to participate and think critically. They need to be taught not to accept things at face value, but to examine things through a process of active mental debate, dissecting each part of the puzzle until it is thoroughly understood. Participative critical thinkers reject ideas that do not add up, accept responsibility when given, share credit with others, admit mistakes they make, and hold themselves accountable for their actions. When personnel are trained with this approach, and the high expectations and level of respect that accompany it, then someday an organization may be built that fully realizes the vision, mission, and potential of the department.

A NEW DAY IS DAWNING

Over the course of his career, this author has seen several attempts at joint training to resolve the issues encountered in the multivehicle crash scenario. Many of these were fairly successful, yet they never fully involved all agencies in the planning stages. Failure to do so usually results in poor scene management and lack of adequate leadership.

One such event was a Joint Commission on Accreditation of Healthcare Organizations (renamed The Joint Commission in 2007)—required hospital disaster drill in 1999. The hospital disaster planning team brought together fire, law enforcement, EMS, 911 (from all three surrounding counties), nursing and EMS students from local colleges, and area emergency management agency (EMA) directors. From a planning perspective, the drill demonstrated that each agency had a willingness to collaborate with the hospital to develop these important drills. However, during the drill, the responses of the various agencies and players demonstrated that there was a lot of work left to do to improve future events. Command was established by the fire department, and EMS established an EMS sector commander to address triage, treatment, and transport sectors. Law enforcement, however, set up its own command and did not participate with the established command system.

The scenario for this drill was twofold. A small explosive device detonated in a hospital stairwell. Ten minutes later, three masked intruders invaded the adjacent nursing home and shot three residents and five staff members. During the incident, hospital security coordinated with the city police department to secure the stairwell after the blast. One of the county sheriff's special operations teams handled the nursing home incident. Neither group communicated with the other responding agencies, nor did they attend the postincident critique. The opportunity to gain valuable working relationships was lost. The lack of true leadership from all agencies most likely caused these failings.

Fast-forward 9 years. Many of these same stakeholders who participated in the hospital drill came together to plan and execute a regional disaster exercise. This idea was formulated by one of the area's county sheriff's department training officers. He then approached the other agencies to develop and execute this multiagency disaster drill to increase area responders' effectiveness.

Staff from a comprehensive group of agencies spent months planning a series of drills as a follow-up to the hospital drill. Participants in the planning included training and supervisory personnel from the sheriff's office, two EMS agencies, two fire departments, the area public health department, volunteer agencies, and the local hospital. Additional participants in the drills included the state bomb squad, state public health officials who used an incident management system (electronic surveillance and tracking), local politicians, school system employees, and, in a few cases, students. These drills focused on a shooter (or shooters; drill participants were not told whether there was more than one armed perpetrator) in a school. Each middle school and high school in the county hosted one drill during the summer for a total of seven drills.

Although these drills were specifically designed to hone the sheriff's department's response to a school shooting, other providers used the opportunity to test and strengthen their competencies by performing their roles simultaneously. The fire departments were charged with command functions; they established the command post, mobile communications center, and unified command. Each public safety agency had a representative at the command post that coordinated communications and responsibilities for his or her respective agency. EMS set up triage, treatment, morgue, and transport areas. At a few of the transport areas, the joint leadership of the represented agencies established a quick-response vehicle that would roll into the hot zone, secure a patient who had been removed from the building, and carry the person to the secure triage area. This occurred using a reserve ambulance driven by a volunteer EMS crew in full body armor, with no fewer than three armed officers (also in full body armor) to protect the EMS crew. At a few of these scenes, although the quick-response vehicle was called for by officers sweeping the building to come and extricate a patient, the vehicle was not released because the command post deemed the mission too dangerous. These drills lasted for 8 hours each day and involved multiple scenarios. This allowed each law enforcement officer, fire officer, and EMS officer to perform the role of sector commander and learn to interact with each other under duress.

At one school, the leadership team placed a powdery substance in an area of the building to see if the officers or the special operations medics accompanying them discovered it. Unfortunately, the officers and medics were not as observant as the leadership team had wished. In response, the leadership team called the local public health department, which sent its response team and enacted the statewide surveillance system. Decontamination processes were practiced and weaknesses in this protocol were observed and addressed.

From a leadership perspective, the best lesson learned during these drills was that both transactional and situational leadership have a role in these dynamic events. Commanders who simply give orders may have the authority to give them even though what they are asking is inappropriate, ineffective, or even dangerous. In the previous drill description, it should be clear that EMS should not have entered the building to retrieve patients because the scene had not been secured. A situational approach called for different actions, but the crews believed they could not be insubordinate and refuse to enter the building or question the order.

THE IMPORTANCE OF CHANGE

One of this author's favorite sayings about the fire service is "200 years of tradition, unimpeded by progress." The expression can also apply to other public safety services arenas. A close family friend, whom the author called Uncle, was the county sheriff for 26 years. He retired from the position more than 20 years ago, and each successive sheriff seems to have had the same approach to leadership as Uncle. They all wanted to stick to their jurisdiction and maintain their authority, just like the previous sheriffs; they were not interested in collaborative relationships with other agencies or in implementing any changes to their office or their profession. Many have refused to participate in joint training with other non–law enforcement public safety agencies, or have only participated in sessions that were mandated. EMS and EMA (formerly Civil Defense) have their own traditions and sometimes also resist change, even though their professions are only several decades old and they are not as steeped in historical perspectives as the older fire and police professions. Change is difficult and often pushes one outside their comfort zone. Many resist change, yet without change one falls behind. Dynamic research and ever-changing methodologies and technologies require

people to adapt and grow, or face stagnation and failure in a profession where lives are on the line in a day's work.

The school shooting drills mentioned previously show how vision and foresight, coupled with a strong commitment to laying the requisite groundwork, can have a lasting effect on joint responses. The training officers of the different agencies charged with carrying out those drills knew that they needed to be able to evaluate NIMS training, coordination of multijurisdictional responses, and collaborative efforts between all responding agencies. These were not easy objectives, considering the lack of coordination between the agencies and various jurisdictions.

Each drill started with instructions from the leadership team on the challenge that lay ahead. However, participants were not told what to do or how to do it. Each agency's training officer gave out that agency's responsibilities. Each either assigned partnered teams and supervisory roles or allowed participating personnel to choose their own roles. Before any drill session started, everyone knew what their roles would be and when they would be called into service throughout the day. After each drill was concluded, teams were encouraged to rest and replenish themselves. After a 20-minute break, the team leaders for each agency performed an initial critique of the session. Numerous key issues were discovered, which were eventually addressed and overcome in successive sessions. During the course of 2 months, interactions between personnel from all agencies took place, valuable lessons were learned, and meaningful and constructive change occurred. Crews from each agency reported better working relationships between themselves and other agencies in the field.

Why do efforts at making substantive change within an organization (or among organizations) often fail? Cultural and personal compacts play a major role. The term "compact" here refers to the relationship between the employer and the employee, as defined by such things as job descriptions, standard operating guidelines or procedures, standing orders, rules, and even law. The word "culture" can mean different things depending on the context. Most commonly, it calls to mind ethnic or religious backgrounds. Yet, organizations usually have their own distinct cultures. Some are run like dictatorships, some like families, and most are somewhere in between. Organizational culture can also vary by region. Some agencies demand that providers work in Class A uniforms, which present an official and formal appearance. Others allow their personnel to dress more casually by wearing a BDU (battle dress uniform) style pants and polo shirts, which reflects a more relaxed and less intimidating appearance. Neither style can be considered wrong; they are just different perspectives on how agencies want their personnel to reflect the department's image. Some departments combine paid and volunteer personnel, which can lead to a culture of competition as the two groups vie for status or recognition. Organizational culture is a powerful force that can affect employees' perspectives, attitudes, and motivation, and the ability of the organization and any of its employees to bring about change.

Leadership Points to Ponder

You have to learn to manage in situations where you don't have command authority, where you are neither controlled nor controlling. That is the fundamental change. Management textbooks still talk about managing subordinates.

Peter F. Druker (2009, p. xiv)

Strebel (1998) describes three common dimensions of personal compacts: (1) formal, (2) psychological, and (3) social. The formal dimension relates to job expectations, such as job descriptions, standard operating guidelines or procedures, protocols, contracts, and other similar documents that detail the performance expectations employers have for their employees. Strebel writes this about the formal dimension:

In return for [an employee's] commitment to perform, managers convey the authority and resources each individual needs to do his or her job. What isn't explicitly committed to in writing is usually agreed to orally. From an employee's point of view, personal commitment to the organization comes from understanding the answers to the following series of questions:

- *What am I supposed to do for the organization?*
- *What help will I get to do the job?*
- *How and when will my performance be evaluated, and what form will the feedback take?*
- *What will I be paid, and how will pay relate to my performance evaluation? (pp. 142–143)*

The reader should ask how these questions affect their commitment to their department.

The psychological dimension refers to how employees commit themselves to the organization's mission and objectives. Subordinates are expected to take responsibility for and carry out organizational objectives and tasks, yet their commitment to meeting these expectations is directly related to the psychological dimension of their personal compact with the organization. Are their personal values and the organization's values similar? Failure to cultivate the psychological dimension results in poor employee performance.

The social dimension is driven by the authenticity and consistency of an organization's culture. Mission and vision statements are the culture the department wants to project to the community and other stakeholders. Employees observe the actions and posture of the administration carefully to see if the vision and mission are reflected in the internal workings of the department, or if they merely serve to project an image to the public. When a mission statement becomes nothing more than public relations, employees are quick to notice. Strebel (1998) writes this about the social dimension:

They translate those perceptions about values into beliefs about how the company really works—about the unspoken rules that apply to career development, promotions, decision making, conflict resolution, resource allocation, risk sharing, and layoffs. Along the social dimension, an employee tries to answer these specific questions:

- *Are my values similar to those of others in the organization?*
- *What are the real rules that determine who gets what in this company? (p. 144)*

Organizational cultures vary widely. However, many organizations in the emergency services practice a time-tested paramilitary model. These cultures are formal in nature and require a high degree of integrity from their personnel. In those organizations that require long stretches of shift work, such as a 24-hour rotation, employees become very social because they consider their peers to be family in many cases.

Leadership Points to Ponder

Only the wisest and stupidest of men never change.
Confucius (from *http://www.thinkexist.com*)

SUMMARY

When in the heat of battle in any situation, command and control of the situation is imperative. The initial scenario demonstrated how people like to play in their own little worlds and practice the leadership (or management) approach for which they were trained. However, as this chapter demonstrates, command and control is not always an appropriate or effective operating principle in all situations. Transactional leadership is a management approach that focuses on control and providing rewards for performing tasks. Like the command-and-control approach, it is an effective tool when used in the appropriate context. Situational leadership is another important addition to the leadership skills toolkit. There is no "one size fits all" theory of leadership. Certain people holding an official role as the "leader" may not be the best people to lead in a particular situation. Many experienced practitioners in the public safety sectors who have been in their fields for many years were taught to manage, but never really to lead.

No matter what one's role, whether manager, leader, or follower, each plays an important part in the organizational structure and effectiveness. Followers need someone to provide direction, leaders need people to follow them, and managers need people to accomplish their tasks. If any of these components fail, the organizational structure is in jeopardy.

Change is occurring in how jobs and personnel are managed. Subsequent chapters provide a glimpse into optional approaches to leadership and how emergency service officers can improve the capacity to manage and lead. Combining management techniques and leadership capabilities helps one manage the logistics of complex disaster scenes, prepare personnel to handle difficult situations, lead units or organizations effectively, and bring out the best in oneself and others.

CHAPTER

Wrap-Up

ACTIVITY

Journal writing is one technique for self-reflection. Approached in the right way, it can be a process of discovery rather than mere reporting. Productive journal writing takes very little time and can be of great benefit. It can be a powerful tool for reflection, self-discovery, problem solving, learning, and integration. Here is how it works:

1. Think about a situation at work with which you are currently struggling or feeling unsettled. (This technique is also good for situations in your personal life.)

2. Write down a set of questions you want to reflect on concerning the situation. Put each question on a separate page, to allow lots of room to write. For starters, try these questions:

   a. What about this situation is uncomfortable or difficult for me?

   b. What did I learn about myself or the situation?

   c. What are all of the possible steps I can think of to take, based on what I have just learned?

3. As you become familiar with this technique, you can vary the questions to accommodate your own needs for personal growth.

4. Decide on a time limit (e.g., 3 minutes per question). If possible, set a timer so you do not have to watch the time.

5. Begin writing. Write about the first question continuously for the allotted time. Write whatever comes to your mind. Do not worry about grammar or punctuation. Just do not stop writing until the time is up.

6. Respond in the same manner, writing continuously, to each question.

7. Try this technique every day, or shift, for a week before you decide whether this approach is a good one for you.

Think about a situation at work that involved your direct supervisor using transactional or situational leadership approaches to handle the situation. After you have reflected on this situation, answer the following questions:

1. Was the incident one where control was required, or could a different approach have been used?

2. If I had been the officer or supervisor, how would I have handled the situation?

3. Would my approach in this situation be considered leadership or management?

4. How did the followers react to the supervisors actions?

5. What can I learn from this incident to better myself as a leader?

Maintaining this journal provides a glimpse of the "you" that most of your peers see and affords you an opportunity to grow as a leader and a person.

REFERENCES

Druker, P. F. (2009). *Managing in a time of great change*. Boston, MA: Harvard Business School Press.

Fiedler, F. E. (1967). *A Theory of leadership effectiveness*. New York, NY: McGraw-Hill.

Followership. (n.d.) In *Mirriam-Webster's online dictionary*. Retrieved from http://www.merriam-webster.com/dictionary/followership

Hersey, P., & Blanchard, K. (1988). *Management of organizational behavior: Utilizing human resources* (5th ed.). Englewood Cliffs, NJ: Prentice-Hall.

Northouse, P. G. (2007). *Leadership: Theory and practice* (4th ed.). Thousand Oaks, CA: Sage.

Strebel, P. (1998). Why do employees resist change? In *Harvard Business Review on Change*. Boston, MA: Harvard Business School Press.

In a Land Far, Far Away

David T. Foster III, Chris Nollette, and Frank P. Nollette

"There's no place like home . . . there's no place like home . . . ". Home is where our hearts are, which is why, when we experience the devastation of a natural or man-made disaster in our communities, we feel like Dorothy being swept away by the infamous tornado in the Wizard of Oz. Leaders forced to deal with catastrophic events would do well to re-examine the message of this classic movie. Having a heart, using your brain, and digging deep for the courage to lead are essential qualities that leaders need now more than ever. However, many of our leaders act more like the Wizard himself. They can be gruff and lack empathy, mainly because they are overwhelmed. Normally, they may be jovial and pleasant, but under stress they react to the pressures in a manner that may remind their staffs of the man "behind the curtain." Leaders must take the time to assess whether they can follow Dorothy's steps down the Yellow Brick Road and lead themselves and their personnel with their hearts, brains, and courage.

INTRODUCTION

This chapter examines leadership under the model of unified command (UC), when multiple responding agencies and jurisdictions with responsibility for an incident share incident management. UC is an element of the well-known Incident Command System (ICS), which was developed in California in the 1970s. More recently, ICS was adopted as a core component of the National Incident Management System (NIMS), which was developed in 2003 by the Department of Homeland Security under Homeland Security Presidential Directive 5. The directive was signed into law by President George W. Bush on February 28, 2003, and called for the development of a nationwide framework that would provide responding partners at all levels (i.e., federal, state, tribal, local, private sector, and nongovernmental agencies) with a common approach to terrorist or natural disaster response.

This chapter explores the challenges of emergency management system leadership in the context of NIMS and UC by examining a disaster scenario and the options and actions of the parties involved. The chapter also revisits leadership approaches discussed in previous chapters and touches on important topics that are relevant to emergency services leaders, including communication, the role of volunteers, ethics, and coping with death and dying.

SCENARIO

A town in the United States has just been hit by an EF4 tornado. The town is devastated. More than 50% of residences are either destroyed or have sustained major damage. The business district has a 70% damage estimate, and all utilities are inoperable. Local emergency services are hampered by the extent of the debris field. State and federal resources have been notified; however, they are most likely 24–72 hours from arrival. Local and neighboring responders are on their own for the time being.

The town is relatively small, with a total population of 1,500 people. Local law enforcement consists of the police chief and six full-time officers. The fire service is an all-volunteer department with a chief who is a career firefighter in another community an hour away. The county has an emergency management director who runs the countywide 911 center. Chaos is rampant as the initial calls for help cannot get through because of damage to the telephone lines and the loss of the main radio tower, which supports the 911 center.

William, the emergency management agency (EMA) director, attempts to organize the few volunteers that arrive, but he cannot communicate efficiently enough to coordinate the response needs. In his frustration, he calls for the mayor to request the National Guard and state police to come in and enact martial law. In notifying all responding agencies of the events taking place and resources needed, there proves to be a major communication challenge. William wants to control all access to the disaster area and every movement of volunteers assisting with this devastating incident. Can he legally do this? Will his actions stabilize the area and aid in the response, or will his actions accelerate the chaos?

COMMUNICATIONS

In 1970, wildfires in California destroyed 700 structures, burned more than a half million acres, and caused 16 lives to be lost (Federal Emergency Management Agency, 2009). As is still common today, the primary weak links that compromised the firefighting and rescue operations were a lack of communication and coordination, not a lack of resources or failure of tactics. The ICS was developed in the 1970s in response to these devastating fires, as a means of addressing those critical weaknesses.

Most people think of communications in terms of radio traffic, satellite telephones, or some other such gear. Yet communication is about much more than just technology. Communication is about transmitting and receiving information verbally and nonverbally. Woods (2006) writes:

> From the moment we rise until we go to bed, our days are filled with communication challenges and opportunities. Unlike other subjects you study,

communications is relevant to every aspect of your life. We communicate with ourselves when we psych ourselves up for the big moments and talk ourselves into or out of various courses of action. We communicate with others to build and sustain personal relationships, perform our jobs, advance in our careers and participate in social and civic activities. Even when we're not around other people, we are involved in communications as we interact with mass media and communication technologies. All facets of our lives involve communications. (p. 3)

As can be seen from this excerpt, communication is the key to everything one does in life. Careers are no exception. To communicate successfully, a person not only has to transmit their messages clearly, but they must also receive and understand the messages of others.

Leadership Points to Ponder

We have two ears and one mouth so that we can listen twice as much as we speak.

Epictetus (from *http://thinkexist.com*)

SCENARIO REVISITED

William's attempts to control the scene, or actually scenes, have done little good. Responders are being pulled into areas and structures by cries for help. Adjoining jurisdictions have sent personnel and equipment, but they are hampered by debris and detained by people waving them down for assitance. Despite William's efforts, there is no command and control in this scenario. Emergency responders have a dilemma on their hands. Does someone take control of responders by establishing a staging area and command center, or do they lead their own responses? According to ICS, the scope and scale of the disaster indicate that William should establish a central command center, known as unified command, with representatives of all responding agencies located there to coordinate the response effort.

William eventually realizes that his initial approach to this incident is not going to work. He is able to get a mobile communications vehicle into the area and is starting to direct all responders who can hear him to come to a single location. He initiates the local emergency response plan and begins to coordinate with other agencies to establish the command center, operations, and logistics. He collaborates with the chiefs of the local emergency services to establish individual branches for fire, rescue, EMS, and law enforcement. Other agencies are also establishing branches to provide leadership and control their respective resources. Public utilities, public health, and volunteer agencies are starting to arrive and request information. Through appropriate training on NIMS, ICS, and UC, responding agencies understand their roles and function and begin to collaborate effectively.

William has now been able to establish a command post and communications. A UC structure is in place. Additional functional units, such as operations and logistics, have been established. Staging, triage, and transport areas have been established. Groups, divisions, leaders, and supervisors are in the process of being established. Temporary communications have been established. Multiple agencies are converging on the area. William has enacted the county response plan and is now functioning as the multiagency coordinator at a field emergency operations center.

APPROACHES TO LEADERSHIP

How does one provide leadership during stressful incidents such as this one? Many emergency service managers are accustomed to using the measures identified as command and control, specifically the "one person in charge" approach to scene management. The initial reaction is to mobilize and control all the resources at one's disposal. This concept and tactic are still valuable resources. However, leadership is more than just management. One needs to know when to use this approach and when to collaborate. What follows is a closer look at some of the leadership approaches and practices that could apply to the scenario.

Collaborative Leadership

Rost described leadership as a process of relationship building with a mutually accepted goal, a definition that certainly applies to the scenario given the number of responding agencies involved and the pressing need for those groups and individuals to work together to address a set of potentially overwhelming and competing demands.

To build the critical relationships that Rost refers to, all stakeholders must be brought to the table long before an incident occurs. Local politicians, fire, law enforcement, EMS, EMA, public utilities, business leaders, area healthcare agencies, and other stakeholders should meet regularly as part of their local emergency planning committees. State and federal agencies should be included as integral partners collaborating in the planning process. NIMS training needs to be provided for all members and their respective personnel who may be called on to respond in an emergency.

What is collaboration? The word originates from the Latin root *collaborates*, meaning to labor together, and has three definitions per Merriam-Webster (Collaboration): (1) to work jointly with others or together especially in an intellectual endeavor, (2) to cooperate with or willingly assist an enemy of one's country and especially an occupying force, and (3) to cooperate with an agency or instrumentality with which one is not immediately connected. For the purposes of this chapter, collaboration is defined as working in conjunction with others to obtain a mutually acceptable course of action and responsibility.

Collaborative leadership emphasizes the involvement of those who have the knowledge and skills to perform relevant tasks. Elected officials, most of whom come from the business world, cannot plan effectively for an emergency response on their own; people trained in all aspects of emergency response need to be part of the planning team. Today's chief officers are often charged with budgetary and political roles over task roles. Despite their excellent professional credentials, many may not be up-to-date on procedures and tactics because of the high-level management priorities they face. Line officers, training personnel, and even street-level personnel from every possible responding agency should be part of the planning process. Other organizations also should be asked to join the local planning committee. The following is a list of potential partners:

- Public and private utilities
- Public and private schools
- Volunteer agencies
- Public health department and area hospitals
- Local builders and contractors
- Building material supply companies

- Heavy equipment operators
- Communications (cellular, radio, ham radio, media, and so forth)
- Politicians (local, regional, state, and federal)
- Businesses (that can provide supplies and services, such as food and water, clothing, housing, and so forth)
- Banks and financial institutions

Preparedness should also include the development of the following resources:

- Plans and protocols
- Interoperability procedures
- Resource support protocols
- Mutual aid agreements
- Operational security measures
- SWOT analysis (strengths, weaknesses, opportunities, threats)
- Functional job descriptions
- Exercise development and review
- Leadership training

Leaders of a collaborative process must set aside political and personal agendas and seek common ground. This is not an easy task, especially when the group of people involved in the planning process is expanded. Each must spend the extra time it takes to build relationships, speaking their minds but taking care not to offend their partners. As anyone who has been through collaborative planning can attest, it is a challenging process that requires patience and sustained effort. However, it is a powerful technique that, when implemented effectively, allows people to optimize the emergency response strategies and prevent response problems before they occur.

Leadership Points to Ponder

Leaders are those who articulate a vision, inspire people to act, and focus on concrete problems and results. [But] collaboration needs a different kind of leadership; it needs leaders who can safeguard the process, facilitate interaction, and patiently deal with high levels of frustration.

Chrislip and Larson (1994)

Situational Leadership

Another *form* of leadership that may now enhance William's success is situational leadership, which focuses on the leader's ability to accurately assess follower maturity and apply appropriate leadership styles to meet their needs. Maturity is defined here as "the ability and willingness of people to take responsibility for directing their own behavior" (Hersey & Blanchard, 1982, p. 151). If William had enacted a planning process long before this disaster and, during that effort, had built relationships with key individuals from responding agencies, he would have a good understanding of how to collaborate effectively with these partners. If one assumes that the personnel resources available to William are competent and well versed in their specific area of responsibility, William should be able to use Style 4 (S4) (see Figure 5-3), or the low-supportive, low-directive style. In using S4, William offers less input as responders carry out their tasks, which is compatible with their maturity level.

Taking this scenario a step further, assume that the person directing the rescue operations and most of the groups performing these functions have been trained appropriately according to NIMS and all of its components. The operations section chief for rescue should be able to apply an S2 or S3 leadership style. Using S2, the chief provides guidance and direction, also referred to as "coaching," and solicits input from personnel operating in the field. With S3, the chief's style is less directive and focuses more on providing the resources that providers need to accomplish their tasks, also referred to as "supporting." An effective leader is able to move fluidly between leadership styles, recognizing that followers have different development levels, or maturity, for different tasks.

Transactional Leadership

Transactional leadership has largely been supplanted by more current leadership theories. It has limited use in multiagency emergency responses and is an approach that William should avoid if possible. The following discussion, from the 2009 Leadership Development Resource Center, presents a cogent explanation of transactional leadership and its shortcomings:

> *The core of transactional leadership lies in the notion that the leader, who holds power and control*

over his or her employees or followers, provides incentives for followers to do what the leader wants. Hence, the notion that if an employee does what is desired, a reward will follow and if an employee does not, a punishment or withholding of the reward will occur. The relationship between leader and employee becomes "transactional"—I will give you this if you give me that, where the leader controls the rewards, or contingencies. (Leadership Development Resource Center, 2009)

Contingent reward is a process in which managers are said to "manage by exception." What this means is that they use an exchange process where the positional leader used something of value as a reward in exchange for a directed behavior. This approach to leadership results in the leader being more concerned with keeping things the way they are. This is not a visionary approach. However, the reality is that it remains a common practice in many organizations today.

Transactional leadership is a management-based process and, although common, lacks the full value of being called leadership as defined in this chapter. The focus is basic management practices of controlling, organizing, and short-term planning. The use of this leadership approach in emergency services revolves more around scene management than personnel management. There are times when a person must use the formal authority of their positions to guide, direct, or even discipline personnel. Therefore, the authors relegate transactional leadership theory to a management theory and not a leadership theory.

Transactional leadership theory involves four dimensions, as follows:

1. **Contingent Reward:** the link of goals to rewards. The leader provides specific, attainable, measurable, and realistic goals for their personnel that can be achieved in a timely manner.

2. **Active Management by Exception:** the transactional leader closely watches their personnel's work, especially violations of standards and rules, and corrects those deviations to prevent errors.

3. **Passive Management by Exception:** the leader only intervenes when they see deviations from standards or performance. This leader usually uses some form of punishment for those deviations.

4. **Laissez-faire:** this approach allows personnel many opportunities to make their own decisions. When the leader takes this approach, the group lacks direction, leading to numerous mistakes caused by lack of guidance on the leader's part.

Using rewards to accomplish goals should rarely be considered in the safety professions, especially during responses to incidents (although it may have its place if used appropriately for rewarding excellence in personnel, teams, and so forth).

Transformational Leadership

Transformational leadership encourages all members of a team or unit to function not only as subordinates within rank-and-file structures, but also as individual leaders. According to Bass (1985), one of the early researchers in this area, transformational leaders are able to *move followers toward higher-order needs* (Northouse 2010, p. 176).

Thus, the police officer, following department policies and procedures, may serve as the sole person responsible for the response to and termination of an incident. The engine company may be the only responder on a call. The officer, although responsible for the actions of the crew, may establish command, yet the person on the nozzle may actually lead the attack and extinguishing of any fire. The EMS crew may be the only unit on scene, with the paramedic in charge of patient care; however, the EMT/emergency vehicle operator is responsible for safely transporting the occupants of the vehicle to and from the scene and assisting the paramedic with direct patient assessment and care while on the scene. Each person, regardless of rank or position in the organization, has a responsibility to provide leadership under certain criteria—at times expected, at times sudden, and at times a necessity for saving the lives of others, including members of one's own unit.

Northouse (2010), one of the field's most respected experts on transformational leadership, writes:

. . . transformational leadership is a process that changes and transforms people. It is concerned with

emotions, values, ethics, standards and long-term goals and includes assessing followers' motives, satisfying needs, and treating them as full human beings. . . . An encompassing approach, transformational leadership can be used to describe a wide range of leadership, from very specific attempts to influence followers on a one-on-one level to very specific attempts to influence whole organizations and even entire cultures. (pp. 175–176)

If William chooses to apply this approach to leadership along with the command-and-control tactics of NIMS, he should be able to successfully guide the responses of initial and subsequent responders.

Leadership Points to Ponder

A community is like a ship; everyone ought to be prepared to take the helm.

Henrick Ibsen (from *http://thinkexist.com*)

ROLE OF VOLUNTEERS

All across the United States and in other countries, volunteers respond to emergency calls on a daily basis. People rely on the professional services of volunteer medical first responders, rescue squads, fire and rescue departments, auxiliary police, emergency management, and others who respond to calls without pay. Similarly, volunteer-based organizations, such as the Red Cross and the Salvation Army, often provide critical relief and assistance after disasters.

Perceptions of volunteers is an issue that leaders must consider, whether leading an organization of full-time paid staff, one with a mix of paid and volunteer staff, or one composed of only volunteers. Too often, volunteers are perceived as being amateurs, people who are merely playing a role, much like an actor on a stage. However, most volunteers today are well-trained, dedicated professionals, closely resembling, if not just like, their paid counterparts. They are typically put through some form of vetting to ensure that their motivations and abilities are compatible with the organization's objectives. Once accepted into the organization (perhaps as a probationary or provisional member), the volunteer undergoes formal training and must pass established oral and written examinations and practical tests or serve

what amounts to an apprenticeship before being fully accredited. Volunteers are expected to contribute both time and effort to the organization and the community, and failure to do so can lead to dismissal.

Years ago, while participating in an on-base theatrical group, one of the authors (Frank Nollette) had the pleasure of working with a member of the group who had wide experience in theater, both as a paid actor and as a participant in community theater productions before joining the Air Force. When someone mentioned that as a group, we would-be actors were amateurs, this individual bristled and lectured us with his perceptions of what we were and what we were doing. His premise was that we were not amateurs but unpaid professionals. Our audiences knew we were amateurs, but that did not excuse us from our obligation to do our utmost to entertain them in as professional a manner as possible. He demanded professional performances of us (particularly when he was director of some of our productions), from learning our lines to our on-stage movements to the many details that make an actor's performance believable. He insisted that we eliminate the word *amateur* from our vocabulary, because he considered it to be a self-defeating term that only served to allow us to rationalize our failures or slipshod performances.

This viewpoint can easily be applied to volunteers in the emergency service community; volunteers are (or should be) considered unpaid professionals. We expect professional performance from paid staff, so why not from volunteers? One cannot expect professional performance from volunteers if they treat them as something apart from the "real" emergency service providers.

Volunteers have an obligation to adhere to the organization's policies, procedures, rules, regulations, and legal requirements, just as do their paid counterparts. Volunteers are likewise subject to discipline for failing to adhere to established norms and may, at the pleasure of the appointing authority, be dismissed. Disciplining volunteers, however, requires even more care than that required for paid organizational members. Unfair discipline (or even the perception that it is unfair) can all too easily result in a loss of many volunteers, despite the leader's best efforts to retain those whose contributions are most valued. If an organization treats its volunteers in a dismissive manner, recruitment and retention of those most needed may prove to be difficult if not impossible.

When people respond to major disasters in and around their communities, volunteers are present. In some communities, the local responders could all be volunteers, and mutual aid agreements may bring these volunteers to neighboring communities. When planning for emergency responses, local entities should include all agencies, paid and volunteer, that are likely to respond during the initial 24–72 hours following an incident.

Leadership Points to Ponder

Emergency preparedness is a team sport.

Eric Whitaker (from *http://thinkexist.com*)

FEDERAL EMERGENCY MANAGEMENT AGENCY IS-240

In December 2005, the Federal Emergency Management Agency released its independent study course IS-240, "Leadership and Influence." The course is a well-written guide for emergency managers that focuses on many aspects of leadership, including facilitating change, building trust, and the need for collaboration and relationship building. It seems that the authors of this course based their approach on Greenleaf's (servant leadership) and Rost's (influence) perspectives of leadership. They immediately set the tone for what successful leadership and influence can look like with the following list of examples:

- Invite other members of an emergency management team to a meeting to discuss common goals.

- Use that meeting as an opportunity to really listen, to learn "where they're coming from" and what they're aiming for.

- Ask for help with or input on a project that will help your community prepare for disasters.

- Speak out to persuade others to accept your point of view.

- Encourage someone else to assume the leadership role in a group.

- Work to establish partnerships with neighboring communities to share resources for prevention, preparedness, response, recovery, or mitigation.

- Recognize the differences among people and draw on the strengths of your organization to prepare for emergencies.

- Marshal local resources to respond during an emergency.

- Demonstrate high standards of honesty, integrity, trust, openness, and respect for others.

The authors also describe three different ways in which people perceive themselves, others, and the challenges before them. They call these perspectives the three lenses of leadership: (1) telescopic (transformational); (2) mid-distance (transactional); and (3) microscopic (technical). Their analysis is that one needs to use both transactional and transformational leadership, with a heavy tilt toward transformational (**TABLE 9-1**). They describe the three lenses as follows:

- Telescopic lens: This lens tends to be transformational. Leaders who look through this lens are more likely to:
  - Establish their beliefs and values and be consistent with them.
  - Determine a course for change in the future and articulate it as a vision.

Table 9-1 Differences Between Transactional and Transformational Leadership

Transactional	Transformational
Leadership is responsive	Leadership is proactive
Works with the organization's culture	Works to change the organization's culture by implementing new ideas
Transactional leaders make employees achieve organizational objectives through rewards and punishment	Transformational leaders motivate and empower their employees to achieve the organization's objectives by appealing to their higher ideals and moral values
Motivates followers by appealing to their own self-interest	Motivates followers by encouraging them to transcend their own interests for those of the group or unit

- Stimulate coworkers and themselves to challenge traditional ways of thinking.
- Develop themselves and others to the highest levels of potential.

■ Mid-distance lens: This lens is usually transactional. leaders who look through the mid-distance lens are likely to articulate standards, policies, goals, and expectations, as well as clear consequences for not meeting expectations.

■ Microscopic lens: Leaders who look through a microscopic lens generally have a laissez-faire style and are focused on specific tasks and details, much like an individual contributor.

Organizing leadership theories into a context that is familiar, such as looking through different lenses in a pair of glasses, helps one to understand key concepts and put them into practice.

ETHICAL CONSIDERATIONS

The most common form of ethics used in emergency services is utilitarianism, which means that the moral worth of an action is based solely on its usefulness in providing happiness or pleasure. In emergency services, this translates to the simple code of "doing the greatest good for the greatest number of people" (Bentham, 1789). Utilitarianism can have extreme consequences for providers in mass causality operations, such as the scenario in this chapter, as the following case study illustrates.

Case-in-Point Abstract

A paramedic who performed triage during a mass casualty call is being questioned by his medical director and mentor about his decision not to treat a 3-year-old child.

A few weeks ago, local emergency services responded to a mass casualty call involving 16 patients. The first unit on the scene immediately established command and began to assign specific roles to each subsequent arriving unit. The first ambulance to arrive on scene was assigned the role of triage. Tom, a 30-year paramedic, began triaging patients. Tom believes in utilitarianism. He was taught that his job is to care for those he can help and not waste limited resources on those he cannot help.

As Tom was assessing the patients, he came across a 3-year-old girl who had an open head injury. She presented with respiration of four to five breaths per minute,

weak carotid pulse, and pupils dilated and unresponsive. Tom also noted that this child had a gastric tube and picline and seemed to have other congenital defects. Tom placed a black triage tag on her, indicating that she was dead, and moved on to the next patient. Tom triaged all patients within 9 minutes of arriving on the scene. All patients requiring immediate medical care were transported off the scene within another 15 minutes. The remaining three patients with black tags and four with green tags (minimal or no injuries) were still on scene awaiting appropriate dispositions.

As Tom and his partner were gathering their equipment, they noticed that a woman had picked up the 3-year-old girl and was running to an awaiting ambulance. Tom hollered at her to stop, but she entered the ambulance and the crew closed the doors and sped away. Tom immediately contacted the command post to determine where the ambulance was going and why they took a patient who had been declared dead. The incident commander assured Tom that he would find out what was going on and get back to him. He then directed Tom to go in-service and respond back to his station. Tom did not get an answer before ending his shift the next morning.

Jim was the EMS Deputy Chief on duty that day and had responded to the same call. Jim assumed the role of EMS sector officer on arrival. He had been informed by the incident commander of the situation with the girl and had followed-up. He discovered that the woman who picked up the girl had been traveling through the area on vacation. She got out of her car, ran up to a medic, and told her that she was a doctor and asked if she could help. The medic directed her to the command post. As she was walking to the command post, she noticed the little girl with the black tag lying there. She felt the girl and determined that she was breathing, had a pulse of two to three beats per minute, and was blue. She immediately yelled to the medic that she had a child in critical condition. The doctor ran with the child to the ambulance, and the medic told her partner to transport the child to the local children's hospital immediately, without awaiting orders or instructions from the scene command structure.

Jim located the ambulance crew and talked to the woman. It turned out that she was a chiropractor, not a physician. She knew nothing about emergency medicine or the structure of emergency scene management. She complained to Jim that it was not ethical to withhold medical treatment from a child who would likely die without it. Jim pointed out that the child had been pronounced dead within 10 minutes of arrival at the hospital and that she had been triaged appropriately. Jim believed in utilitarian ethics too and believed that, at best, medical care would have only briefly prolonged this child's life and, at worst would have taken critical care away from other patients who needed it more.

Sharon is the medical director of the local EMS system and has trained most of paramedics in the area. Sharon received a call from the chiropractor, stating that she was looking for the family of the child and was going to tell them that the paramedics allowed the girl to die by incorrectly tagging her as dead. She demanded that Sharon fire those incompetent emergency medical technicians for allowing the child to die. Sharon has called a meeting with Jim and Tom to discuss the issue.

The following dialogue takes place.

Sharon: *Hi Tom and Jim, please sit down. I received a call from a Dr. Shorty. She was the doc on the mass causality call y'all ran a few weeks ago. She is seeking the family of the little girl you triaged, Tom, to encourage them to sue you and us for allowing her to die.*

Tom: *Doc, I did just as you trained me to . . . .*

Sharon: *Hold on, Tom, I need to see your scene documentation. I have known you too long to think that you would not have done as you were taught.*

Tom: *I did not do any documentation since I did not transport any patients.*

Jim: *Doc, I kept the call log of all EMS activity on the scene.*

Sharon: *Okay, Jim, then I need you to provide that to me along with every patient care report of all patients who were transported from the call.*

Jim: *I can get that for you.*

Tom: *Doc, I did exactly what I was supposed to. I assessed every patient there and determined that I had three patients whose injuries were beyond their viability. As for the little girl, I knew I had five other critical patients and four immediate potential life threats and only six ambulances available for transport. You taught me to do the best for the most, did you not?*

Sharon: *Yes I did, but I need to know that your reasoning for tagging her black was based on sound, reasonable, critical thought. Did you . . .*

Tom: *Doc, that's BS. You know me. I did what was best for her. She had an open head injury, plus she had a g-tube and a pic-line. She was also the only one who most likely would not have benefited from surgical intervention. The probability of her surviving was extremely low.*

Sharon: *Okay, but each of you has a duty to act. Sometimes you have to do things that may violate the ethical perspectives of other people. However, you must base those decisions on sound reason. Can you tell me that if this were to go to court, a jury or even a judge would understand that we place black tags on people who we think will die but are actually still alive?*

Tom: *I don't care what they think. We have to make life-and-death decisions on an almost daily basis. We do decide at times who is viable and who is not. I would have put all my effort into treating her appropriately if she had been my only patient, or one of only a few patients and we had had enough ambulances to care for everyone.*

Jim: *Doc, this child had several congenital defects and was probably in constant pain. That is no way to live. Her parents were probably keeping her alive to satisfy their own guilt or needs, not hers. After all, even if she had survived, could she have lived a full and happy life? I think not. Tom did exactly right, in my opinion.*

Sharon: *Jim, do you mean to tell me that if this were your child, you would not have a duty to care for her?*

Jim: *Maybe I would, but she wasn't my child or Tom's, and Tom had to do what was best for everyone at the scene, not just her.*

Sharon: *So, what I am hearing from you, Tom, is your reasoning to not tag her red was that, based on your assessment, you determined that her injuries, along with her vital signs, coupled with her previous medical problems, made her untreatable? Is that your reasoning?*

Tom: *Yes, ma'am, it is.*

Sharon: *Do you believe you had a duty to provide anything else for her? How about comfort measures?*

Jim: *Doc, come on, comfort measures? On a disaster call?*

Sharon: *Jim, do we not teach y'all that you have a duty to provide a patient with comfort measures where appropriate?*

Tom: *Doc, Jim is right, we do not do that, and you know it, especially in a disaster situation. Why are you grilling us on this? We were only doing as you taught us. I feel betrayed.*

Sharon: *Okay, guys, I feel that you did exactly as you should have. However, I have to be comfortable with the reasoning behind your actions. Our attorneys are going to question me about whether your actions were not only legal, but ethical also. Each of us has different views of what is ethical. Many people, especially those in the press, will most likely try to make this a case of you playing God, Tom, even though you feel that you did nothing unethical.*

I agree with you, but I have to be able to convince our counsel that you provided quality treatment, based on reasonable standards of care, and that your actions met our society's definition of ethical behavior.

Jim: *So where do we stand here?*

Sharon: *Get me all the documentation on the call so I can review it and ensure that everyone followed the appropriate protocols. Once I am satisfied that every action was based on what the crews were taught, and knew to do, then I will take our stance to risk management and our attorneys so they can prepare for any possible questions or litigation.*

Thanks, guys, for your time today. Overall, my preliminary findings are that you did exactly what you were supposed to. It also appears that you did an excellent job under the circumstances. If anything else comes up with regard to this case, I will let both of you know. Have a good day.

Jim: *Thanks, Doc, see ya later.*

Tom: *Thanks, Doc. I have a better understanding now of where you are coming from. I feel better about the whole situation. Talk to you later. Bye.*

How often have actions seemed right to one person but wrong to others? Ethical and moral views can conflict with those of others, and understanding ethical theories

and standards helps when one is faced with defending their actions.

Death and Dying

Physicians and other healthcare professionals have little training or education regarding death and dying. "By any standard one chooses, medical schools in the United States fail to provide even adequate education in the care of the dying" (Hill, 1995, p. 1265). A random survey by Dupont and Francoeur (1988) of schools of medicine, nursing, and social work "revealed no evidence of a consensus of the need for death education for health professions, no evidence of systematic development of course content or approach and no evidence of any attempt to integrate training and facilitate collaborative team care in this area" (p. 33).

A study by Schoenberg and Carr (1972) involving healthcare professionals concluded that in the area of death and dying, "inadequate education in the management of the terminally ill probably represents one of the greatest failures in professional education today" (Mermann, Gunn, & Dickinson, 1991, p. 35). Although this study was done more than 28 years ago, the accuracy of this conclusion is still being cited by experts in the area of death and dying. If physicians and other allied health professionals lack the training and education to deal with death and dying issues, then those in public safety have certainly been left out of the equation, despite the fact that they deal with death and dying on a daily basis.

The conversation between Sharon, Tom, and Jim underscores the importance of this issue. When the medical director questioned the decision not to work a young patient who later died, the paramedics contended that they did the "best for the most" and had to make some hard decisions. The medical director is caught in a bind; she trained and educated these men to make these tough decisions but finds herself having to defend the legality of their actions. The comments that paramedic Jim made, "That is no way to live" and "Her parents were probably keeping her alive to satisfy their own guilt or needs, not hers," may be seen by some as a realistic view of the world, whereas others may see this as cold and indifferent. The other paramedic, Tom, states, "We have to make life-and-death decisions on an almost daily basis." The stress of making these difficult decisions while dealing with the hard reality of limited resources can leave healthcare providers feeling frustrated and at times hopeless.

The reality is that EMS professionals lose far more critically ill or injured patients than they can save, an emotional challenge they often face with little or no training. Without such training, the psychological pressures of the job can quickly become overwhelming. The cumulative effects of witnessing death on a large or small scale, day after day, can lead to persistent physical, emotional, and psychological problems that can affect not only the individual, but also the individual's patients, coworkers, and family members. In the absence of comprehensive education on death and dying, many professionals resort to unhealthy coping mechanisms, such as denial, suppressing emotions, dehumanizing patients, labeling episodes as unavoidable, humor, and failing to talk with loved ones about their experiences on the street, none of which addresses the underlying problem. All public safety professionals should seek training on death and dying to help them deal constructively with the substantial stresses and demands of the job.

Leadership Points to Ponder

Any man's death diminishes me, because I am involved in mankind; And therefore never send to know for whom the bell tolls; it tolls for thee.

John Donne (from *http://thinkexist.com*)

CONCLUSION

The role of an emergency services leader is complex and multidimensional. Success in crisis management does not come solely from one's abilities, but also from building relationships that allow one to influence outcomes effectively. When a person possesses the appropriate technical skills, coupled with the ability to influence decision making in a positive, ethical, and virtuous manner, both under duress and during normal day-to-day operations, then they are well on their way to becoming an exemplary emergency services leader.

CHAPTER

9

Wrap-Up

■ ACTIVITY

Take a moment and list 10 values that you have; think about these carefully. Values can best be defined as your beliefs. Once you have listed 10 values, trim the list down to 5 values that you cannot live without.

When leaders reflect on their values (beliefs), they can better understand the guiding force that shapes their ethics, otherwise known as "behavior." Although values can change, so can ethics (behavior). Many leaders say they value those who work for them. When is the last time that you said thank you to those who work for or with you?

Many leaders say that they value their family. When is the last time you really spent quality time with your family, away from the texting and email that seem to find their way on vacation with all of us?

■ REFERENCES

Atkinson, P. (2009). *Political correctness*. Retrieved from http://www.ourcivilisation.com/pc.htm

Bass, B. M. (1985). *Leadership and performance beyond expectation*. New York, NY: Free Press.

Bentham, J. (1789). *An introduction to the principles of morals and legislation*. Oxford, UK: Clarendon Press

Chrislip, D. & Larson, C. (1994). *Collaborative leadership: How citizens and civic leaders can make a difference*. San Francisco, CA: Jossey-Bass.

Collaboration. (n.d.) In *Merriam–Webster's* online dictionary. Retrieved from http://www.merriam-webster.com/dictionary/collaboration

Dupont, E. M. & Francoeur, R. T. (1988). Current State of thanatology education in american health professions and an integrated model. *Loss, Grief & Care, 2*, (1–2), 33–38.

Federal Emergency Management Agency. (2005). *Leadership and influence*. FEMA Independent Study Program, Emergency Management Institute. Retrieved from http://training.fema.gov/EMIWeb/IS/

Federal Emergency Management Agency. (2006, March 26). NIMS Basic, FEMA 501-1. Retrieved from http://www.oema.us/files/FEMA_501-1.pdf

Federal Emergency Management Agency. (2009). *NIMS and the Incident Command System*. Position paper. Retrieved from http://www.fema.gov/txt/nims/nims_ics_position_paper.txt

Hersey, P., & Blanchard, K. (1982), *Management of organization behavior: Utilizing human resources* (4th ed.). Englewood Cliffs, NJ: Prentice Hall.

Hill, T. P. (1995). Treating the dying patient: The challenge for medical education. *Archives of Internal Medicine, 155*(12), 1265–1269.

Leadership Development Resource Center, Better Leaders-Better Workplaces. (2009). *What is transactional leadership.* Retrieved from http://work911.com/leadership-development/faq/transactional.htm

Mermann, A. C., Gunn, D. B., & Dickinson, G. E. (1991, January). Learning to care for the dying: A survey of medical schools and a model course. *Academic Medicine, 66*(1), 35–38.

Northouse, P. G. (2010) *Leadership: Theory and Practice,* (5th ed.), Thousand Oaks, CA: Sage

Politically correct. (n.d.). In Merriam-Webster's online dictionary. Retrieved from http://www.merriam-webster.com/dictionary/politically+correct

Schoenberg, B., & Carr, A. (1972). Educating the health professional in the psychosocial care of the terminally ill. In B. Schoenberg & A. Carr (Eds.), *Psychosocial aspects of terminal care* (pp. 3–15). New York, NY: Columbia University Press.

Woods, J. T. (2006). *Communication mosaics: An introduction to the field of communications* (4th ed., p. 3). Belmont, CA: Thompson-Wadsworth.

10

Downtime

David T. Foster III, with excerpts from Chris Nollette

It is possible to impart instruction and to give commands in such a manner and such a tone of voice to inspire in the soldiers no feeling but an intense desire to obey, while the opposite manner and tone of voice cannot fail to excite strong resentment and a desire to disobey.

The one mode or the other of dealing with subordinates springs from a corresponding spirit in the breast of the commander. He who feels the respect which is due to others cannot fail to inspire in them regard for himself, while he who feels, and hence manifests disrespect toward others, especially his inferiors, cannot fail to inspire hatred against himself.

MG John M. Schofield,
Address to the United States Corps of Cadets, August, 11 1879
(from *http://regimentalrogue.com/quotes/quotes_discipline1.htm*)

■ INTRODUCTION

This chapter examines leadership in nonemergency situations. How should the officer lead when command and control is not needed (leadership as an influence relationship)? Leadership of a unit, crew, or shift from within the rank and file is also considered. These line personnel may be referred to as "unofficial leaders" because they are the ones the other line personnel actually listen to and follow.

This chapter explores how personal perspectives can hinder relationships with others. These perspectives are based on personal biases and can lead to conflicts. A leader's lack of political savvy or poor emotional skills may lead to controversy in his or her agency.

■ CHAPTER SCENARIO

You are working in a fire department that runs emergency medical services (EMS) transport. Your station houses one basic life support engine company and an advanced life support ambulance. Your station officer, Captain Buford,

is a 30-year veteran of the fire service who is known for his autocratic style of leadership. Captain Buford is an extremely intimidating individual. He refuses to accept EMS as a function of the fire service. The rest of the crew consists of Kevin, a 4-year firefighter and a paramedic assigned to this engine; Steve, the senior firefighter and an EMT who has been with the department for 16 years; William, a 20-year veteran of the fire service who is the fire apparatus operator of the engine company; and Thomas and his partner Marty, both seasoned veterans of fire and EMS with 21 years' experience each as firefighters and paramedics. Thomas and Marty have worked on engines, rescues, and the ambulance. Thomas also carries the rank of captain in the EMS division.

As part of the station routine, the crews do housekeeping details in the morning and in-station training during downtime during the day. Captain Buford is constantly complaining that "those ambulance drivers are never here to do their share of the work and are not carrying their weight around here." The tension between Captain Thomas and Captain Buford is now at a breaking point. Captain Buford insists that this is his station and he will see to it that the ambulance drivers help maintain it.

A NEW DAY IS DAWNING

Dealing with the daily routines of emergency services is usually much different than operating on the emergency scene. Having one person in charge in an emergency is often essential. If a scene becomes overwhelming or multiple agencies are operating jointly, one needs to consider a unified command structure. However, during downtime, a command-and-control approach to leadership can be counterproductive. As this chapter illustrates, leading from a position of respect is much more effective than leading from a position of authoritative control.

> ### Leadership Points to Ponder
>
> *Do you wish to be great? Then begin by being. Do you desire to construct a vast and lofty fabric? Think first about the foundations of humility. The higher your structure is to be, the deeper must be its foundation.*
>
> Saint Augustine (from *http://thinkexist.com*)

Consider the following situation, where a police officer working a scene demonstrated a great understanding of leadership influence, as witnessed by the lead author of this chapter. The incident was a motor vehicle crash, and the sole occupant of the vehicle was highly inebriated. When the rescue crew got the occupant extricated from the vehicle, they saw that he had a small laceration on his left cheek. He refused medical treatment and was placed in a patrol car to be transported to the jail. By the time the transporting officer got the driver to the booking room, he was pretty upset with the officer. EMS was called to the jail to reassess the individual. Shortly after the arrival of EMS, the initial officer from the call came in. He sat down with the subject in custody and, in a calm voice and with a lot of respect, explained what was going to happen and described the booking process. He insisted the individual get medical care. Once the ambulance left, this officer sat down with the transporting officer and held an impromptu class on dealing with subjects under the influence. He explained how any slight insult or offending tone can trigger rage in an inebriated subject and easily lead to a hostile and hazardous situation. What did he do that was different from what most officers would do? He showed compassion, respect, and empathy for the subject in custody and the other officer. All are characteristics of leadership. He very easily could have come in, barked a few orders, and controlled the situation (or escalated it) through command. Instead, he chose to act through influence.

SITUATIONAL LEADERSHIP APPLICATION

Situational leadership is a theory that can be applied in a multitude of situations. This section expands the theory into a practical application, which the reader can use in various situations. So the question now is: How can a person practice leadership when they are programmed to manage? Start by realizing that situational leadership is one of many viable options. If a person tries to command his way through each situation, then his is are merely dictating, not leading. Situational leadership (Hersey & Blanchard, 1969) proposes that leaders should adapt their style to their followers' development level (or maturity), which is based on how ready and willing the follower is to perform required tasks (i.e., their competence and motivation). The focus here is that optimal leadership varies from one situation to another. No single approach works best for every situation (**FIGURE 10-1**).

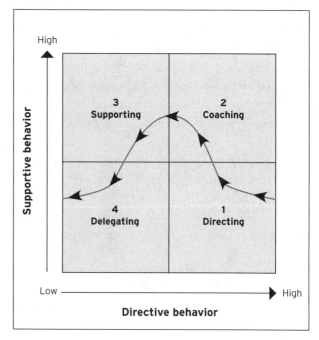

Figure 10-1 Situational leadership.

There are four leadership styles (S1–S4) that match the four development levels (D1–D4) of followers. The four styles suggest that leaders should put greater or less focus on the task in question or the relationship between the leader and the follower, depending on the developmental level of the follower. Northouse (2007) writes the following regarding situational leadership: ". . . leadership is composed of both a direction and a supportive dimension, and each has to be applied appropriately in a given situation" (p. 91). A deeper look at what these levels mean follows.

S1 **Telling/Directing** refers to a leader who has high task focus and low relationship focus. This leader defines the roles and tasks of followers and supervises them closely. This approach is applicable to the rookie as he or she is transitioned from a training environment to work on the street. They may have the knowledge; however, they may also lack the experience of applying that knowledge.

S2 **Selling/Coaching** refers to a leader who has high task focus and high relationship focus. This leader still defines roles and tasks but seeks ideas and suggestions from followers. Decisions remain the leader's prerogative, but communication is much more two-way. This approach is better geared for situations that allow for collaboration. Consider a multiagency drill, where the crew members are preparing for their roles. The officer may ask for ideas and suggestions on how to accomplish the team's tasks.

S3 **Participating/Supporting** refers to a leader who has low task focus and high relationship focus. This leader leaves most decisions and the allocation of tasks to followers. The leader facilitates and takes part in decisions, but control is with the followers. This approach may apply when the team members are all well-seasoned personnel and highly competent. A good leader wants to see their team members succeed and possibly even exceed what the leader has accomplished. Allowing team members to make decisions and learn from their mistakes and success builds from this approach.

S4 **Delegating** refers to a leader who has low task focus and low relationship focus. This leader is still involved in decisions and problem-solving, but control is fully with the followers. They decide when and how the leader is involved. Although not the most desirable of approaches for emergency services personnel, a leader could use this approach in training sessions. This allows personnel to apply their knowledge in controlled situations without input from the formal leader. This could prove essential in emergent situations where something happened to the formal leader and a crew member had to step up and take charge.

Likewise, the competence and commitment of the follower can also be distinguished in four quadrants:

D4 **High Competence/High Commitment** refers to followers who are experienced at their job and comfortable with their ability to do the job well. May even be more skilled than the leader.

D3 **High Competence/Variable Commitment** refers to followers who are experienced and capable but may lack the confidence to go it alone, or the motivation to do it quickly and well.

D2 **Some Competence/Low Commitment** refers to followers who may have some relevant skills but are not able to do the job without help. The task or the situation may be new to them.

D1 **Low Competence/High Commitment** refers to followers who generally lack the skills required for the job but have the confidence or motivation to tackle it.

Hershey and Blanchard (1969) indicate that leadership style (S1–S4) must correspond with the follower's developmental level (D1–D4). In this model, the leader is the person who adapts, not the follower. It is assumed that this approach leads to followers' growth and development, builds better relationships between leaders and followers, and leads to better outcomes.

Leadership Points to Ponder

Always do right. This will gratify some people and astonish the rest.

Mark Twain (from *http://quotationspage.com*)

TODAY'S EDUCATED WORKFORCE

The personnel of today are better educated and have more technical expertise than those of previous eras. Many departments now require an associate or bachelor's degree for hiring or promotions. Workers bring with them new skill sets that enhance their ability to think critically in high-stress situations. They respect the chain of command during an emergency. However, they most likely balk at the old style of management by intimidation. For leaders, formal rank or not, it is imperative to recognize the talents of the people around them and build relationships based on respect, confidence, and loyalty.

Leadership Points to Ponder

You do not lead by hitting people over the head—that's assault, not leadership.

Dwight D. Eisenhower (from *http://thinkexist.com*)

SCENARIO REVISITED

The scenario that started this chapter showed an officer who leads through control and intimidation. He lacks an understanding or acceptance of the principles of contemporary leadership. He has not accepted the department's new role as a prehospital medical provider. He still believes that everyone should contribute equally to station work, regardless of call volume. He fails to acknowledge that the EMS crews run between 70% and 80% of the incoming calls.

CONFLICT

Dealing with this type of regimented, nonyielding individual is difficult at best. Confrontations most likely escalate the tensions and do not resolve the issues. According to the Merriam-Webster Dictionary (Conflict, n.d.) conflict is defined as

1: *FIGHT, BATTLE, WAR <an armed* conflict>
2a: *competitive or opposing action of incompatibles: antagonistic state or action (as of divergent ideas, interests, or persons)*
2b: *mental struggle resulting from incompatible or opposing needs, drives, wishes, or external or internal demands*

3: *the opposition of persons or forces that gives rise to the dramatic action in a drama or fiction*

synonyms see DISCORD

In the scenario, definitions 2a, 2b, and 3, or a combination of these could be used to describe what is occurring between these officers. However, 2b may best describe the animosity that exists between the two captains. Captain Buford's wishes and Captain Thomas's are much different. This could be the result of differences in generation, education, perception, or experience, among other possibilities.

Johnson and Johnson (2009) suggest that we are all "unique individuals with separate wants, needs, and goals"(p. 368). Wants are desires for something. Perhaps Captain Buford desires the old days before EMS intruded on his department. Needs are necessities for survival. Is it possible that Captain Buford feels threatened by another person of the same rank being in his station and is therefore lashing out as a survival mechanism? A goal is an ideal state of affairs. Captain Buford's goal is probably something that he envisioned for the department, or himself, and has been working toward for many years. Combine these three elements and he probably feels threatened and even intimidated by the growth and changing dynamics of the department. It is possible, even likely, that the department has outgrown him.

Conflict can be dealt with by applying one or more strategies. One can force the issue, which usually results in a poor outcome for all involved. One can withdraw, choosing not to continue a confrontation, which is sometimes the best choice. It may seem as if one has surrendered, and sometimes that is fine. Smoothing over the issue is another approach, or sometimes people just agree to disagree. If the goal is of little importance, yet the relationship is highly important, this approach saves the relationship and assists the other person in achieving their goal. Compromising allows both parties to come to a mutually acceptable position on the matter. This approach works best when both parties are motivated to resolve the issue constructively with a minimal investment of time. When both parties have a strong desire to achieve their goals and maintain their relationships, then they will engage in true problem solving. With this approach, participants peel back the layers of their conflict to identify the underlying problems that may have been hidden under superficial issues. In the end, both parties achieve their goals as fully as possible, compromise where necessary, and resolve the tensions and bad feelings that surfaced during the conflict. However, this approach requires a substantial commitment of time and effort, as well as difficult moves, often perceived as risky, such as revealing one's true feelings while not being sure that the other person will offer the same degree of candor.

An alternative approach is for Captain Thomas to build a risk coalition. A risk coalition, also called a risk agency, is a group of like-minded individuals with shared views. Think of this as something similar to union leaders who represent members of an organization; these individuals are usually not formally represented. They represent themselves with the help of influential members of the organization's power structure and outside stakeholders. Should Captain Thomas choose this route, he must address issues as they relate to other members of the department. The other station personnel may feel that Captain Buford has belittled them, shown a lack of respect for their contributions to the unit, limited their advancement, or any number of other things that could be undermining performance and morale.

POLITICAL SAVVY

Influence is an essential part of leadership. Influence refers to the change in a target agent's attitudes, values, beliefs, or behaviors as a result of influence tactics. Political savvy is essentially a form of influence.

Political savvy is a skill that anyone serving in any organization, especially a government agency, needs to develop. Personnel in government agencies do not operate independently. Their work is subject to immediate and unforeseen change because newly appointed or elected officials may decide to take public services agencies in different directions. An individual with political savvy fully understands the internal and external forces impacting her department or agency and is able to use this understanding to further her own goals and those of the organization. Like emotional intelligence, political savvy helps leaders influence others and bring people of varying styles and perspectives together to build consensus on key issues.

The word "politics" brings about visions of saying what people want to hear, often with little regard for being authentic or truthful. However, these negative connotations are not part of the word's actual meaning. "Politics" is derived from the Greek words *politikos* and *polis*, meaning citizen and city, respectively, and the French word *savoir*, meaning to know or understand. Political savvy is one's ability to know or understand the people in the community. Those who have political savvy can navigate effectively through complex organizational and interpersonal challenges because they listen to others, learn about what is important to them, and take their needs into consideration. Above all, they treat people with respect. In contrast, the person who is purely political focuses on personal gain without regard for the interests of others. It is important to understand the difference. Political savvy is a useful tool for effective leadership. However, being political can do irreparable damage to one's standing with colleagues and, ultimately, to one's career.

EMOTIONAL AND SOCIAL INTELLIGENCE

Captain Buford's emotions are palpable; he has no problem in sharing the deep-seated resentment and anger that he feels toward the EMS unit and crew. However, feeling and displaying emotions is not the same thing as emotional intelligence. In fact, Captain Buford's posture and behavior demonstrate precisely the opposite: a lack of emotional and social intelligence.

There was a time where fire departments spent most of their time fighting fires. As education and fire prevention methods have become more effective, fire departments find themselves with fewer fire response calls. The reality is that in many communities, EMS has eclipsed the original mission of the fire department. With EMS calls now accounting for approximately 70%–90% of a department's call volume, fire departments are no longer in as much jeopardy of downsizing. Instead of viewing this change in a positive light, Captain Buford seems to be facing the new reality with a mixture of fear, resentment, and anger, and he has let his negative emotions take control. How could he approach the situation more constructively? It is useful to look at the components of emotional intelligence and see how they could serve Captain Buford and his department. It is important to understand at the outset that emotional intelligence is not an innate skill; all people can benefit from studying the emotional intelligence recipe.

The Emotional Intelligence Recipe
Self-awareness: Cornerstone

Captain Buford would benefit from an honest assessment of where his anger and frustration are coming from. He may find that they stem from a concern that he may be replaced. After all, EMS gets most of the calls, so it is understandable for him to feel that they must be more vital to the mission of the department. Or they may be caused by feeling marginalized and not having the control and authority he once had; EMS is not Captain Buford's area of expertise, so he no longer feels like the most experienced and knowledgeable person in the room, as he once did when surrounded by junior firefighters. Or, unbeknownst to the crew, factors in his personal life may also be causing him stress and exacerbating the tension. At this point in the scenario, we certainly do not understand all the contributing variables in the situation, and it is likely that Captain Buford does not either. Introspection is a productive first step for him to take in resolving the conflict. Without self-awareness, one is handicapped in any endeavor, personal or professional.

Managing emotions

Emotions are a wonderful and important part of being human. In fact, brain research has shown that emotions helped humans survive and evolve. When early humans encountered large predators, for example, the rush of fear triggered the fight-or-flight response in the sympathetic nervous system, a reaction that remains essential for managing immediate and severe threats to well-being. However, emotions can also be damaging. Because Captain Buford feels threatened, he often operates in a state of heightened negative emotions when dealing with the EMS professionals in his department. He is prone to outbursts and often does not think about the impact his words might have before he speaks. He would benefit greatly from learning that thinking acts as a brake on one's emotions. Police officers know this well and use it to their advantage when they separate people at a scene and begin to talk them down. The more the officers talk, and the more suspects engage with them, the more quickly the strong emotions drain away. Thinking is

critical to saying and doing the right things—something Captain Buford has not explored up to this point.

Motivation

Captain Buford must develop his emotional intelligence by motivating himself and taking responsibility for is own actions. The blame game is old and outdated and has never been effective, but it is easy to do. Change, however, is never easy, especially when it calls into question leaders' authority and makes them feel insecure about themselves and about what lies ahead. It is easier for Captain Buford to blame EMS for disrupting his department than to find a way to work with them. Captain Buford would need a great deal of motivation to confront the situation constructively and seek a positive resolution.

Empathy

Empathy is critical to building and maintaining emotional intelligence. Empathy means being able to identify with and understand someone else's situation and feelings, commonly referred to as "putting yourself in someone else's shoes." Empathy requires taking the time to put people above process, focusing on the individual for a moment rather than the mechanics of the job. Empathy is a critical part of being a good leader and person. When one makes people feel they have been listened to and understood, one earns their trust. In addition, valuable insight into situations is gained, which is essential for navigating the complex dynamics of an organization, especially during times of change. Both Captain Buford and the other members of the fire and EMS units would benefit from using empathy in this conflict. Starting from a position of trying to understand another person reduces tension, suspicion, fear, and other negative emotions and helps avoid the damaging impact of a hostile confrontation.

Relationships

Dealing effectively with decision making, consensus building, change, and especially conflict is challenging for any leader. This challenge can become nearly impossible for someone who does not have relationships with colleagues and other stakeholders. Put simply, relationships are critical for the success of individuals, teams, and especially leaders. The ability to develop working relationships with others forms the basis of social intelligence. Rather than building relationships with members of the EMS unit, Captain Buford has distanced himself with his belligerent demeanor. If Captain Buford had been trained in the importance of social intelligence, he might have taken the time to build relationships with the EMS personnel who joined the fire department. Those relationships would have helped everyone involved handle the changing dynamics of the unit more constructively.

CONCLUSION

Leadership at the station should look a lot different from leadership at the scene of an emergency, although the issues faced during downtime can be as challenging or, in some ways—as Captain Buford's situation illustrates—perhaps more challenging than the toughest 911 call. For the scenario to be resolved, the root causes of the tension and animosity need to be uncovered. Is Captain Buford misunderstood, threatened, or just plain set in his ways and refusing to change? These issues must be identified and resolved through the application of problem-solving methods. Because it seems unlikely that Captain Buford has the skills to initiate and manage this process, it may take intervention from those of higher authority in the department. Administration may also choose to use a nonbiased mediator to resolve this issue. As a leader, always consider all options for dealing with conflict, and try to resolve issues systematically, compassionately, and above all ethically. One's skills in guiding personnel during nonemergent situations will no doubt be tested as rigorously as skills in directing them through a time of crisis, and will be an important component of success as an emergency services leader.

10

Wrap-Up

ACTIVITY

Mentoring others is critical for any good leader, and to be an effective mentor, one must also be mentored properly. Good leaders seek out a mentor. Great leaders seek the talents and support of a variety of people to help them grow in different areas and learn different perspectives. In what areas of your personal and professional life could you benefit from the help of a mentor? Can you identify individuals you could turn to for mentoring in these areas?

1. Do you need a mentor to help you in your personal life, including family issues like spouse and children?

2. Do you need a financial mentor?

3. Do you need a mentor who has great interpersonal and intrapersonal skills?

4. Do you need a mentor to show you how to relax and de-stress after a hard day?

5. Do you need a mentor who can help you in developing professional relationships with your employees?

6. Do you need a mentor to hold you accountable for your leadership style and professional growth?

REFERENCES

Conflict. (n.d.) Merriam-Webster's online dictionary. Retrieved from http://mw4.m-w.com/dictionary/Conflict

Hersey, P. & Blanchard, K. H. (1969). *Management of organizational behavior—utilizing human resources.* Upper Saddle River, NJ: Prentice Hall.

Johnson, D., & Johnson, F. (2009). *Joining together: Group theory and group skills.* Upper Saddle River, NJ: Pearson.

Northouse, P. G. (2007). *Leadership: Theory and practice* (4th ed.). Thousand Oaks, CA: Sage.

11

The Challenges of Being the Chief

David T. Foster III

In Flight of the Buffalo (Stayer & Belasco, 1993), the authors describe two different types team leadership. One type resembles the style used by wild buffalos. One lead buffalo dictates every move the herd makes. In nature, buffalos are loyal creatures that have been known to follow their leader into precarious situations without regard for their own safety. Native Americans exploited this loyalty during buffalo hunts by killing the leader first, thus creating confusion in the rest of the herd.

Geese offer a different approach to leadership. As the flock flies the characteristic "V" formation, leadership changes when the need for different skills arises. One goose might be adept at locating food, while another is expert at navigation. Each goose takes turns leading the formation based on the situation, needs, and environment of the entire group. Research has shown that during the flight, the wings of each bird create an uplift for the bird behind it. This enables the entire wedge of geese to fly much farther than a bird flying alone. As they fly, the trailing geese encourage their leader by honking. They are also loyal creatures. If one bird becomes ill or injured, two others follow it to the ground and protect it until it expires or recovers. Whichever occurs, the geese then return to the flock to continue their journey.

As a leader, are you more like a buffalo or a goose?

INTRODUCTION

This chapter examines the pressures and challenges faced by leaders in emergency services, and it offers several models and strategies with an emphasis on Bolman and Deal's (2003) model of reframing that leaders can use to avoid and overcome these issues. Autocratic and servant-oriented leadership styles and their consequences are contrasted. Finally, how misguided leadership may result in rank-and-file personnel bypassing the established hierarchy to drive change on their own by forming a risk coalition is examined.

SCENARIO

Chief Mac has been the chief of police in a major city for the past 15 years. He came up through the ranks in the uniformed division, detective division, and training division over a 30-year career. He held the rank of deputy

chief of training for almost 20 years before his promotion to chief of police. Many of his officers know how he became the head of training and disagree with the move. Mac was severely injured one rainy night at a motor vehicle crash. When he arrived on scene, he found a car with a woman inside yelling for help. As he approached the car, he failed to scan the scene for hazards. He grabbed the door handle and was immediately knocked to the ground. He had not seen the downed power line touching the car. He was fortunate to survive. Afterward, the administration moved him to the training division, because he was not physically able the return to the streets. As a training officer, he was known to be brash, unyielding, and autocratic. However, in public, he was a social butterfly. Everyone who did not have to work for him thought the world of him. His ascent up the ranks was mainly because of his charisma and the "good old boy system."

During his tenure as chief of the department, Mac played political games for promotions. He surrounded himself with people who supported him, and he rewarded their loyalty with favoritism. As other area departments advanced with the times by embracing rapidly changing technologies, Chief Mac adamantly resisted change and kept the department in his comfort zone. He held the budget down for years by not requesting equipment, appropriate pay increases, or technologic advancements. His lack of progressive thinking and his failure to keep abreast of these changes allowed him to hold the budget at bay. Not purchasing new equipment or taking advantage of federal grants led to a static budget that pleased the politicians, who embraced Chief Mac's approach to holding down the department's costs. By the time he retired, the department was considered 20 years behind the times.

Chief Mac's word was final. If a person tried to advocate for advancement of the department, they were labeled a troublemaker. Many of the older officers with years of service and ties to the community suffered through his tenure. Junior officers, who were more mobile than the older officers, remained in the department just long enough to gain state certifications, then departed for other agencies. Late in Chief Mac's career, the rank and file became restless and staged a confrontation. This occurred mainly via several media blogs. Some expressed concern to local politicians, but this concern was met with skepticism.

> ### Leadership Points to Ponder
>
> *Nearly all men can stand adversity, but if you want to test a man's character, give him power.*
>
> Abraham Lincoln (from *http://thinkexist.com*)

After a lengthy nationwide search, Chief Mac was replaced with Chief King, one of the department's deputy chiefs and Mac's right-hand man. King is just as autocratic as his predecessor, yet he lacks Mac's charisma. Riding the coattails of his mentor, he has built a strong bond with the local politicians, and his promotion signifies the political comfort zone. If city officials had wanted to grow and improve the department, they would have chosen an outside candidate with fresh ideas and methods. The promotion of Chief King sends the strong message that the politicians wish to perpetuate the ways of the previous administration.

However, King's personnel do not trust him to carry the department forward. To do this, he needs to substantially increase the department's budget for equipment, vehicles, training, and payroll. Department officers and line personnel currently make over 20% less than most of their peers in neighboring jurisdictions, and they have demanded higher pay. Presenting his first budget to the political body will reveal the degree to which King intends to fight for bringing his department to current standards. Chief King also would be well served by developing promotional processes based on candidates' abilities, knowledge, and past performance. Any appearance of favoritism or discrimination undermines his integrity and diminishes his already compromised standing with his staff.

LEADERSHIP IN PROFESSIONAL PUBLICATIONS

During the past several years, professional publications for emergency service disciplines have published articles on leadership. A review of these articles reveals that in many, the term "leadership" is applied to those with positional authority, such as officers charged with command and control, scheduling, purchasing, task assignment, discipline, and public information. These articles discuss how leaders should manage their departments and personnel, without regard for the role of line personnel (followers) in leadership. However, not every article embraces the positional approach to leadership. Several articles in 2009 relate leadership to the needs of department personnel. One such article describes a partnership between a mental health professional and the chief of a department to develop a leadership training program based on Robert Greenleaf's servant leadership model (B. J. May, 2009). The premise of the project is that learning to lead by serving increases buy-in to the mission and vision of the department and builds the self-worth and morale of its personnel.

Another article also focuses on followers. The author asks who is best qualified to determine a leader's ability: peers, managers, or subordinates. The author concludes that subordinates (line personnel) are best suited to provide this perspective (Alyn, 2009). However, as the author acknowledges, officers (managers) typically conduct performance evaluations. It seems that if one wants to determine the effectiveness of leadership in officers, then subordinates, not supervisors, should conduct or at least contribute to performance evaluations for their commanding officers. This is not a new concept. Many businesses use what is known as the "360 performance appraisal," where an employee's performance is evaluated by the direct supervisor, peers, direct reports, and the individual's internal and external stakeholders. Although the primary goal of this process is to evaluate performance, the results are often used to identify strengths and weaknesses for the purpose of targeting professional development.

Although approaches such as this are by no means common in emergency service disciplines, leadership that focuses on the relationships between line personnel and officers is gaining greater acceptance in these professions. An example of this is a regional award given each year to an emergency medical services (EMS) director as determined by the agency's personnel. The nomination must come from someone other than upper administration, and the winner is determined by a questionnaire filled out solely by employees.

SERVANT LEADERSHIP

In the 1970s, Robert Greenleaf explored leadership as service, a model he called "servant leadership." Greenleaf's emphasis was on leaders nurturing their followers. Followers have concerns, perspectives, and needs to which leaders should be attentive. As leaders focus on the needs of their followers, they empower the followers to develop, both as professionals and as individuals.

In our scenario, Chief King is well advised to address the needs of his followers. For King to engage in servant leadership, he needs to reinvent his approach to running the department. He is on the proverbial hot seat with his personnel. They are expecting him to change the organizational culture of autocratic leadership, political patronage, and stagnation that has existed for years. Advocating for better pay and benefits for his personnel would be a good first step for King toward servant leadership and would show them that he cares about their welfare and morale. Remember, though, that a budget increase would likely be a tough sell with the politicians, whose appointment of King indicated their desire for business as usual.

King should consider building his administrative team around this concept of service. As the chief of police, King has a responsibility to address the needs of all stakeholders. For example, what inequities exist in the community with regard to policing? Were certain neighborhoods or areas ignored by the previous administration? Using the servant-leader philosophy, King could approach the citizens of high-crime areas about

partnering with the department to establish a community policing advocacy group. Northouse (2007) writes the following regarding serving communities:

> *In becoming a servant leader, a leader uses less institutional power and less control while shifting authority to those who are being led. Servant Leadership values everyone's involvement in community life because it is within community that one fully experiences respect, trust and individual strength.* (p. 349)

When studying the facets of servant leadership, it becomes clear that researchers and advocates of this leadership process fully embrace the ethical perspectives of leadership. The leader–follower relationship is the starting point of ethics as advocated by some scholars. By taking an ethical, servant approach to leadership, one becomes a steward of the vision of the organization. This vision is greater than any one person, including oneself.

Leadership Points to Ponder

The first responsibility of a leader is to define reality. The last is to say thank you. In between, the leader is a servant.

Max De Pree (from *http://thinkexist.com*)

FIVE GUIDING VALUES

In the summer of 2006, during the National Association of EMS Educators Course, one of the instructors related a story about a fellow EMS educator's ethics lecture for his emergency medical technician (EMT) class. The educator challenged his students to identify five values that could guide them on their journeys to becoming EMTs and throughout their careers. They came up with the following guiding values: (1) respect, (2) integrity, (3) compassion, (4) empathy, and (5) accountability. After sharing this list with colleagues, the educator discovered that the acronym could be rearranged to spell out "I CARE" (Le Baudour & Nollette, 2006).

Integrity

Compassion

Accountability

Respect

Empathy

The acronym "I CARE" is an excellent way to frame a code of ethics. These five words, or values, are discussed next in detail.

Integrity

When one deals with another person's property, belongings, or life in situations of great stress, acting with integrity is of the utmost importance. The word "integrity" comes from the Latin *integer*, meaning number or whole unit. Integrity is, first of all, about being one, or being whole. Integrity is about having a sense of one's own basic commitments, sticking to them, and sticking up for them. Like other virtues, integrity is deeply ingrained in one's character through long years of training and commitment. Such virtues cannot be turned on and off like a water spigot. Rather, they are deeply entrenched habits; they are part of who we are.

Compassion

Compassion is considered a virtue in many philosophies and is an important element in the world's major religions, including Christianity, Judaism, and Islam. Although attributes such as integrity and accountability play a role in many professions, compassion has special relevance for EMS professionals. Compassion combines sympathy for another person with a desire to help—a condition that should be considered the foundation for action in emergency services.

Accountability

Accountability means being responsible for one's actions. To be responsible is to accept judgments, acts, and omissions (refusals or failures to act) as one's own burden where appropriate, in whole or in part. Although superiors often apply accountability externally, the most powerful form of accountability rests within each person, as he strives to reach the ethical and professional standards he sets for himslf.

Respect

Respect is a powerful ethical value. German philosopher Immanuel Kant brought the notion of respect to the center of moral philosophy for the first time (Saunders, 2004). "Kant created a moral system that was open to everyone capable of reason, regardless of their religious beliefs. The bedrock of his system was respect for the dignity of all human life" (Ciulla, 2003, pp. 94–95).

When this author is teaching first responders, EMTs, paramedics, or other healthcare providers, whether they are from EMS, fire, or law enforcement, he stresses that they should respect patients as if they were one's mother, father, wife, husband, or other family member. This may not always be easy, especially in situations requiring command and control, but it serves one well when performing the job most of the time.

Empathy

Empathy means trying to imagine what someone else is feeling and sharing in those emotions. Empathy is essential in the field of emergency services, because the nature of the profession is dealing with people who are often in great emotional distress. Being able to meet such distress with empathy is a powerful way to help victims not just psychologically, but also physically because stress plays an important role in physiological response. Another model that uses five guiding principles for ethical leadership is presented by Northouse (2007) (see **Figure 11-1**).

There is no single set of values one should adopt to the exclusion of others. Many powerful elements of ethical leadership are contained in both the Northouse model and the I CARE model, and one can no doubt think of others. Ethics and values did not guide Chief Mac during his tenure, and one can see the resulting damage to the department. Chief King has an opportunity to lead the department in a new direction, based on higher standards, but to do so, he needs a solid foundation of guiding values, such as the ones presented previously.

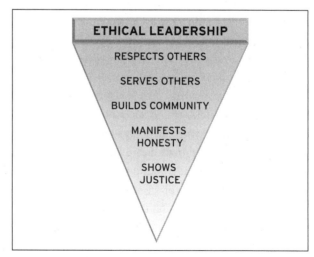

Source: Adapted from Northouse, 2007, p. 350.

Figure 11-1 Guiding values of ethical leadership.

REFRAMING DEPARTMENTS FOR THE FUTURE

Perception is a powerful thing. How people see, or perceive, the world around them is driven by many factors: family influence (or lack thereof) during the formative years; teachers and coaches; friends and peers; religion; culture; and others. Faulty or incomplete perceptions can drive a person to make bad choices, both personally and professionally. Perhaps the reader has had the experience of writing off a new acquaintance based on a poor first impression, only to find after getting to know the person that the first impression was completely wrong. Faulty perception by managers and leaders plays an important role in organizational failures.

In their widely read book, management experts Bolman and Deal (2003) describe "the curse of cluelessness," which they say results from flawed perception, and they provide a set of four frames, or ways of looking at situations, that people can use to improve and broaden their perspective. They write:

Learning multiple perspectives, or frames, is a defense against thrashing around without a clue about what you are doing or why. . . . When the world seems hopelessly confusing and nothing is working, reframing is a powerful tool for gaining clarity, regaining balance, generating new options, and finding strategies that make a difference. (pp. 21–22)

An examination of these four frames in detail, as defined by Bolman and Deal (2003), shows how they could help Chief King move his department in a more positive direction. Each frame addresses a different facet of an organization's identity:

The structural approach focuses on the architecture of organization—the design of units and subunits, rules and roles, goals and policies. The human resource lens emphasizes understanding people, their strengths and foibles, reason and emotion, desires and fears. The political view sees organizations as competitive arenas of scarce resources, competing interests, and struggles for power and advantage. The symbolic frame focuses on issues of meaning and faith. It puts ritual, ceremony, story, play, and culture at the heart of organizational life. . . . The symbolic lens, drawing on social and cultural anthropology, treats organizations as temples, tribes, theaters, or carnivals. It abandons assumptions of rationality prominent in other frames and depicts organizations as cultures propelled by rituals, ceremonies, stories, heroes, and myths rather than rules, policies, and managerial authority (pp. 16, 21).

The frames have four key dimensions, which appear in **TABLE 11-1**. Think of these dimensions as the four sides of a window frame; each side helps make up the full frame, or view.

Table 11-1 The Four Frames of Leadership Model

	Structural	Human Resource	Political	Symbolic
Metaphor for organization	Factory or machine	Family	Jungle	Carnival, temple, theater
Central concepts	Rules, roles, goals, policies, technology, environment	Needs, skills, relationships	Power, conflict, competition, organizational politics	Culture, meaning, metaphor, ritual, ceremony, stories, heroes
Image of leadership	Social architecture	Empowerment	Advocacy and political savvy	Inspiration
Basic leadership challenge	Attune structure to task, technology, environment	Align organizational and human needs	Develop agenda and power base	Create faith, beauty, meaning

Source: Adapted from Bolman and Deal, 2003, p. 18.

Metaphor for Organization

The metaphor for the structural frame is a factory, where products are assembled the same way through a repetitious process, or a machine, which functions through a rote process. The mechanics of an organization, such as the organizational structure, job descriptions, and formal procedures, are an important underpinning of its successful functioning. In the human resource frame, the organization is seen as a family unit, with its obvious emphasis on people. Like families, organizations are composed of people who bring their own distinct histories, perspectives, goals and priorities, strengths, and weaknesses. Successful organizations can identify and harness individuals' strengths and make people feel good about the work they do. The political frame casts the organization as a jungle: relentless, competitive, and marked by the struggle to survive in a landscape of threats and limited resources. In their most interesting metaphor, for the symbolic frame, Bolman and Deal (2003) liken the organization to a carnival, theater, or temple, thus evoking an atmosphere that includes polar opposites ranging from jovial and fun to reverent and subdued.

Central Concepts

The central concepts of the structural frame are straightforward: rules, regulations, policies, goals, objectives, and the many tasks that are required to accomplish the organization's mission. The human resource frame focuses on the needs, skills, and relationships of its people. The political frame is about jockeying for position and power, driven by conflict and competition for the scarce resources; it is departmental politics, pure and simple. The key concepts in the symbolic frame are the organizational culture: What does it mean? What are the organization's rituals, ceremonies, and stories? Who are its heroes?

Image of Leadership

The structural frame is viewed as social architecture. How do leaders create service-oriented organizations or create the space for people to act on the things that matter to them? The human resource image is empowerment, which Bolman and Deal (2003) direct toward the people in an organization. Empowering people means to shift power from a title or an individual at the top of the hierarchy to the people under this power. This gives them an equal say, or at least the power to speak freely about decisions that affect them. In the political frame, advocacy leads the way. Leaders advocate for their people, missions, and social causes. In the symbolic frame, the image of leadership is inspiration to the organization. Good leaders inspire their people to think critically for the greater good of the organization and to solve problems creatively.

Basic Leadership Challenges

In the structural frame, leaders focus on aligning the organizational structure to its tasks, technologies, and environment. When the structure is aligned with the organization's key components, the "machine" functions smoothly. The human resource leadership challenge is to optimize the match between the department's needs and those of the employees, allowing each to flourish to its potential. In the political frame, the leader's priority is to develop the organization's agenda and solidify a power base because, as Bolman and Deal astutely observe, "you need friends and allies to get things done" (2003, p. 220). Finally, in the symbolic frame, the basic leadership challenge is to create faith, beauty, and meaning for the organization as a means of tapping into people's deep-seated desire to participate in an endeavor that is greater than the sum of its parts.

SCENARIO REVISITED

Applying Bolman and Deal's (2003) model to this chapter's scenario, the first and most obvious recommendation is for Chief King to look at his organization through the four frames to gain perspective, understanding, and knowledge of his situation. A breakdown of some specific objectives for each of the frames follows.

Structural

The previous chief kept the department under-resourced in terms of equipment and technology. Any investment Chief King makes in these areas may require new tasks, procedures, and roles. King needs to look through the structural frame to ensure that his organization's "machine" works smoothly after its mechanical overhaul. In addition, Chief King should consider shifting from an autocratic structure to a more democratic one.

Human Resource

This frame represents both a major challenge and a huge opportunity for Chief King. Morale is low, young recruits are leaving the department, and there was already some effort by the rank and file to undermine the previous chief. If Chief King seeks meaningful, positive change in his department, the human resource frame is an ideal place for him to start. However, his first major human resource challenge, that of increasing salaries, is a tough one. Nonetheless, Chief King could find some initial success in the human resource frame by empowering his crew to assist him in reframing the department. This would be a significant cultural shift that would appeal to people's desire to contribute and have an impact beyond their daily tasks.

Political

The past administration, of which King was a part, was driven by this frame and was corrupted by the power of belonging to the "good old boys club" of local politicians and officials. It was learned from Chief Mac's tenure that powerful political forces are arrayed against change, including any potential effort by Chief King to increase the allocation of resources for his department. Chief King also faces equally powerful pressure for change from within his department. Careful examination of his situation through the political frame can help Chief King walk the tightrope of these competing interests and find compromise that appeases both sides. It is not enough to placate the established power base. To find any lasting success, Chief King needs to take the political risk of advocating for his officers. Because the political frame is so critical in this scenario, the next section takes a more in-depth look.

Symbolic

According to Bolman and Deal (2003), this frame helps leaders "create faith, beauty, meaning." Looking through the symbolic frame at the current organization, one sees the failures cultivated over the years by Chief Mac, Chief King, and others in their inner sanctum. The department is in the doldrums; it lacks pride, cohesion, and spirit and is instead filled with rancor and discontent. There are many complex elements to this condition, some more difficult to improve than others. Chief King could start by using one of the simplest and most time-tested tools in

the leadership toolkit: listening. If Chief King listened carefully to how members of his department feel about their situation and their ideas for change, he would increase their faith in his commitment to them and begin the process of rebuilding relationships with them. There are many other creative ways Chief King could use this frame, but listening is a powerful starting point.

EXPLORING THE POLITICAL FRAME

Drawing on the work of numerous contributors, Bolman and Deal (2003) propose four key activities that a manager or leader needs to engage in when addressing organizational change through the political frame.

1. Set an agenda: This is the leader's vision for the department and how that vision is to be accomplished. Chief King should develop a team of departmental advisors from all ranks, age groups, and cultures representative of the department to create this vision and the strategies for accomplishing the vision. Chief King could view this as the Super Bowl of his career. Going into budget hearings, to name just one example, with a well-developed game plan based on how other teams have performed in the past is essential. If Chief King is not ready to challenge and counter each move the politicians make, each step could be his last.

2. Map the political terrain: According to Bolman and Deal, "A simple way to develop a political map for any situation is to create a two-dimensional diagram mapping players (who is in the game), power (how much clout each player is likely to exercise), and interests (what each player wants)" (2003, p. 217).

3. Network and form coalitions: Chief King should not only build the advisory team (coalition) discussed in step one, but he should also network with other department chiefs. Researching their pay scales, capital equipment plans, and other budgetary issues provides valuable insight into current best practices and where others have found success (or failure). Learning from others is a valuable tool. Few people are the first to walk the path on which they tread. Someone, somewhere, has walked the same path, has fought the same battles, and has the scars to prove it. There is no

sense in reinventing something that has proven successful, unless a newer approach could lead to better success.

4. Bargain and negotiate: This step can be directly linked to transactional leadership: one gives in return for getting something of value.

Bolman and Deal (2003) recommend an approach developed by conflict resolution gurus Fisher and Ury called "principled bargaining," which includes the following four strategies:

1. Separate the people from the problem. As Bolman and Deal write, "The stress and tension of negotiations can easily escalate into anger and personal attack" (2003, p 213). When people are taken out of the equation, this counterproductive force is neutralized.

2. Focus on interests, not positions. Failure to do so may blind one to better alternatives to achieving the goal.

3. Invent options for mutual gain. Mind traps and groupthink are detrimental to successful outcomes. Developing multiple alternatives increases the likelihood of success.

4. Insist on objective criteria. One must have current and accurate data, which is essential to developing objective and measurable criteria. Some questions that must be answered are: What are the substance and procedure involved? What are other justifications paying for like services? What is the cost to the public?

Chief King is at a crossroads. He can choose to maintain the status quo or risk his career by standing up ethically for his men and women. The options are many, complex, and fraught with risk. Formulating a sound strategy for dealing with the political component of this situation must be a priority for King if he is to take on the challenge of change and weather it successfully.

Leadership Points to Ponder

Your reputation and integrity are everything. Follow through on what you say you're going to do. Your credibility can only be built over time, and it is built from the history of your words and actions.

Maria Razumich-Zec
(from *http://www.leadershipnow.com*)

RISK LEADERSHIP

Risk leadership empowers midlevel and lower-level employees of any organization to challenge the formal base of authority and drive needed change themselves. According to Brungardt and Crawford, "most true change agents are not the recognized leaders, but rather, are the lower-level energetic employees of the organization" (1999, p. 31). They contend that when employees lack confidence in an organization's leadership and direction, they can empower themselves to change course and steer the organization in a different direction.

Leaders of this kind of change are often bright, talented, dedicated, and enthusiastic individuals who can articulate an alternative vision or path for the organization and enlist the support of others in their mission. They are usually well respected by their peers, even though they may have been with the department for only a short period.

To accomplish their goals of forcing change and transforming their departments, these change agents must join with others, aggregating their lower-level power to create a force formidable enough to take on the status quo. These individuals work together out of a shared sense of purpose, with the common goal of helping the organization reach what they believe is its true potential. Brungardt and Crawford (1999) refer to such a coalition as a "risk agency." The approach takes its name from the risk inherent in such a strategy. Understandably, those at the top of the organizational hierarchy may not react favorably to the efforts of lower-ranking employees to circumvent their authority. Hence, risk leadership requires skill, commitment, and the determination to prevail against what may be challenging circumstances.

In the public safety professions, it is the line officers, shift officers, supervisors, EMTs, medics, firefighters, and other personnel who must carry out department mandates. If they are not included in the formulation of those mandates, then the likelihood of department leaders gaining full buy-in to their missions is slim. It is these frontline personnel whose energy and initiative make departments succeed.

CONCLUSION

There are many challenges to being the "boss." When a person tries to appease those he or she answers to, they tend to ignore those they rely on to accomplish their mission. Chief Mac built up a great deal of political capital with those elected to run his jurisdiction. However, he alienated most of his personnel by not providing them the personal and professional resources they needed to accomplish their jobs. Although he was challenged by the rank and file, it seems that they failed to build a strong coalition from middle managers, a key upper manager, and influential community stakeholders.

The choice of Chief King to be the new chief carried several political undertones. First and foremost is the politicos' message to keep the status quo intact. Next is the fact that they believe someone outside would attempt to make radical changes, thus creating more controversy than their choice. This is not to say that Chief King cannot be successful in advancing the department, although it will require him to rebuild trust with his personnel and community stakeholders. By using the reframing process and being aware of his own weaknesses and the challenges he faces, he can be successful.

Many pitfalls challenge the leader of any organization. These include outside influences, rules and regulations, organizational culture and structure, ethical and moral obligations, and personal and professional risk. Regardless of one's role, position, or level of authority within an organization, they still have people to whom they are accountable. These may include elected officials, municipal managers, regulatory agencies, employees, and the communities they serve. Employees can make their leaders accountable in several ways. They can challenge and confront leadership to make positive change. They can vote with their feet and leave the organization. They can also use their political clout to advocate for removal from office. Whatever method they choose, if they build the approach properly, they can force change even if the administration refuses to adjust. Personnel are the main resources. Failing to treat them as such can have ramifications that may not be to the liking of administrators.

To lead an organization to a new way of thinking, learning, and doing, one first must have faith in their own visions. One usually does not get it right the first time, so there is a need to experiment, evaluate, reflect, and collaborate with those who have done it before and learn what does and does not work. Then, and only then, can a person fulfill their journey with positive, lasting results that empower them and their followers.

11

Wrap-Up

ACTIVITY

Using a department or organization with which you are familiar, create a diagram of the department's administrative chain of command. Then expand the diagram to include people and stakeholders to whom the head of the organization is accountable. Finally, rank these people according to who has the most influence over the organization. For each influential stakeholder, answer the following questions:

1. How can this person/group influence the department head?

2. How much influence does this person/group actually have, and what are the main ways they wield that influence?

3. Does their influence seem to follow one of the leadership theories discussed in this text, or is it more about control and coercion?

4. If you were the head of this organization, could you work effectively to build alliances with each influential stakeholder to create a mutually acceptable approach to leading the organization?

REFERENCES

Allen, S., & Hartman, N. (2009). Sources of learning in student leadership development programming. *Journal of Leadership Studies, 3*(3), 6-16.

Alyn, K. (2009). Great leaders: Take input from their followers. *Firehouse Magazine*, July, 2099. Retrieved from http://www.firehouse.com/topic/other/great-leaders-take-input-their-followers

Bolman, L. G., & Deal, T. D. (2003). *Reframing organizations: Artistry, choice and leadership* (3rd ed.). San Francisco, CA: Jossey-Bass.

Brungardt, C., & Crawford, C. B. (1999). *Risk leadership: The courage to confront and challenge.* Longmont, CO: Rocky Mountain Press.

Ciulla, J. (2003). *The ethics of leadership.* Belmont, CA: Wadsworth/Thomson.

Le Baudour, C., & Nollette, C. (2006). *The "I-CARE" story*. Retrieved from http://www.icarevalues.org/story.htm

May, B. J. (2009). Marketing ICS: Servant leadership in the fire and emergency services. *Firehouse Magazine*, December 2009. Retrieved from http://www.firehouse.com/topic/leadership-andcommand/marketing-ics-servant-leadership-fire-and-emergency-services

Northouse, P. G. (2007). *Leadership: Theory and practice* (4th ed.). Thousand Oaks, CA: Sage.

Sanders, J. (2004). Honor among thieves: Some reflections on professional codes of ethics. *Professional Ethics, 2*(3–4), 83–103.

Stayer, R.C. & Belasco, lA. (1993). Flight of the buffalo: Soaring to excellence, learning to let employees lead. New York, NY: Warner Books

12

Ever-Changing Roles

David T. Foster III

On January 6, 1919, at his home in New York, Theodore Roosevelt died in his sleep. Then–Vice President Marshall said, "Death had to take him sleeping for if Roosevelt had been awake, there would have been a fight." When they removed him from his bed, they found a book under his pillow. Up to the very last, Teddy Roosevelt was still striving to improve himself. The mark of a great leader is constant learning and growing.

INTRODUCTION

Regardless of historical practices in the emergency services professions, officers at all levels also are followers. They are accountable to someone else in the administrative hierarchy. This applies to everyone, including line officers, training officers, chiefs, and politicians.

This chapter focuses on team building and conflict management as keys in developing effective training programs. We explore these subjects by reviewing the work of several women who have ascended to leadership roles in their respective departments. The perception that women are weaker leaders than men has been proven inaccurate in numerous studies of women managers and leaders. This is explored in depth, looking at how women have become successful in all emergency services disciplines. Regardless of gender, leaders have a responsibility to their personnel, and that responsibility is to train them to be better, smarter, and more successful, much as a parent does with their children.

SCENARIO

United County is a large county serving a population of more than 400,000 residents. It has a daily transient population of 750,000 because of a large manufacturing base. The emergency services of the county have consolidated their resources to establish a countywide public safety training center. This center has partnered with a regional college to provide training and postsecondary education courses for its personnel.

The new director of the United County Public Safety Academy, Christina Jones, is a veteran firefighter and paramedic. Like many of her peers, she first obtained an associate's degree in fire science. After several years in the fire service, she was promoted to chief of training for the fire department and then advanced up the ranks through the emergency medical services (EMS) sector. During this time, she earned a bachelor of science in EMS management. Jones later went on to obtain a master's degree in public administration and a doctorate in education. Although she has no direct experience in law enforcement, her father is a former deputy chief of the county police department. This upbringing afforded her a great deal of insight into the workings of law enforcement.

Chief Jones has ascended the ranks and managed to break through the "glass ceiling" faced by so many women in the profession. It has not been an easy journey, but Jones persevered and prevailed against many obstacles with great determination. However, her success came at a price that, unfortunately, is all too common for women in leadership positions, especially in EMS. Throughout her career, she was seen as an outsider, the "Queen B" (not the nice "B" word), an "ice princess" because of her distance and apparent coldness, and other unflattering characterizations. However, Chief Jones is a great educator. She had the strongest academic credentials of all the candidates for this position. Union County's administrators are confident that she is the most qualified person to bring the vision of the jurisdiction together. They are counting on her to build a top-tier reputation for the new academy.

Chief Jones's responsibilities include managing the academy and its budget, and building and maintaining relationships with the college and other stakeholders. She is also responsible for providing instructional development for the more than 20 instructors of the academy. The academy provides all initial training (certification and licensure) for law enforcement, fire, EMS, and emergency management agency (EMA) personnel. In addition, the academy provides in-services, continuing education, and personnel development courses for all the agencies. Through a partnership with the college, courses are offered for the county's emergency services personnel as part of an associate's or bachelor's degree. A new initiative for Jones is to establish partnerships with area high schools to provide instructional and career development courses for students interested in pursuing these fields postgraduation.

CHIEF JONES'S CHALLENGE

Chief Jones's greatest challenge is to bring the various agencies' training officers on board with the mission of the new academy. Some instructors are resentful that their respective training centers were consolidated. One instructor made the statement that they had no business trying to be a college; his personnel did not need degrees to be excellent field providers. When he was asked by Chief Jones to clarify his comment, his response was, "It's simple: degrees are something found on a thermometer!" With a climate of resentment, self-interest, and skepticism among the instructors, Jones has her work cut out for her.

ALONE AT THE TOP

The fact that Chief Jones is the only woman on the instructional staff and one of very few women in leadership among the different agencies is likely to hamper her efforts to unite this group of resentful and, in some cases, hostile instructors. Even though she has support personnel who are women, she is alone at the top—a situation faced by many women in leadership positions, especially in the field of emergency services.

In the 2000 census, as reported in a 2008 study by the International Association of Women in Fire and Emergency Services titled "A National Report Card on Women in Firefighting" (Hulett, Bendick, Thomas, & Moccio, 2008), women made up 3.7% of first-level firefighters and just 2.9% of first-line supervisors. The survey also found that nearly three and a half times the percentage of women serve in non-frontline roles, such as fire inspection and investigation (16.6%), compared to fire suppression (4.8%). Among departments that responded to the survey, the only job where women had greater representation than men was firefighter paramedic, with women making up 36% of the ranks compared to 30.5% for men. According to the report, "In some cases, these differences reflect individuals' preferences, while in other cases they are involuntary. Either way, they are likely to limit perceptions of women as full members of the working team, as well as prospects for promotions" (p. 9).

Although the numbers remain small, there are signs that they are trending upward. In 2010—women held the top spot in 15 Fortune 500 companies compared to 10 in 2006—small numbers, but a 50% increase. Women ran for president and vice president of the United States in 2008. In 2004, the San Francisco Fire Commission approved Joanne Hayes-White as the next chief of the San Francisco Fire Department.

PERCEPTIONS OF WOMEN IN LEADERSHIP

Despite these advances, women still face formidable obstacles in their climb to the top. Research shows that women in leadership positions are more likely to be looked on by their male counterparts as either coddlers or dictators. Lips (2009) writes about this limited dichotomy of perceptions to which women in leadership roles are often confined, adding other pejorative descriptions to the ones above:

> It appears that the acceptable scripts for women in powerful public political roles are still rigidly defined and easy to violate—by being too "pushy" or too "soft," too "strident" or too accommodating, too sexless or too sexual. It seems all too easy for women leaders to run afoul of their constituents or their colleagues by deviating from the narrowly-defined set of behaviors in which cultural femininity overlaps with leadership.

This phenomenon that Lips and others have observed puts many women leaders in a catch-22 position, particularly in emergency services: either they are seen by men as not tough enough to command respect in leadership roles or, if they seek to prove their toughness, they face the withering criticism that Chief Jones has had to endure of being too tough.

Interestingly, the stereotypically male style of macho, heavy-handed leadership is at odds with the more contemporary leadership models discussed elsewhere in this book, such as Greenleaf's servant leadership, Burns' transforming leadership, and Rost's postindustrial theory. These approaches focus on such elements as relationship-building, teamwork, mutual respect and trust, service to others, providing a supportive environment, and listening to followers' needs; all things that, ironically, fall closer to the stereotypical priorities and behaviors of women than men.

Although researchers have tried to nail down specific gender differences in leadership styles, it seems that no gender is more suited to lead than the other.

> In a meta-analysis, Eagly and Johnson (1990) found that contrary to stereotypic expectations, women were not found to lead in a more interpersonally oriented and less task-oriented manner than men in organizational settings. These differences were found only in settings where behavior was more regulated by social roles, such as experimental settings. The only robust gender difference found across settings was that women lead in a more democratic, or participative, manner than men. (Northouse, 2007 p. 266)

All people are different from each other in one way or another, whether gender, personality, education, skill set, or some other trait of physiology or character. Women are just as capable as men to lead, and women, like men, practice a range of leadership approaches, from transactional to transformational. For Chief Jones to be successful in building her team, she would be well served by using a relationship-building influence process (Rost) along with a focus on service (Greenleaf).

A PERSPECTIVE FROM TWO WOMEN IN FIRE AND EMS LEADERSHIP

The following looks at what Kim Ransom, Deputy Chief of Douglas County, Georgia, Fire/EMS Department, and Brenda Beasley, RN, BS, EMT-P retired of Alabama, two of many highly capable women in emergency services, have to say about their experiences as they rose to leadership roles.

When You Started in Your Career, How Many Women Worked in Your Agencies?

> *Deputy Chief Ransom: I think I was number five in the field, none of them on fire apparatus. I started on an ambulance and eventually transferred to a fire truck, and at the end back to an ambulance.*

> *Ms. Beasley: When I entered the EMS profession, there were only about six women in this state who were involved in EMS education, and many of those women were nurses teaching EMS. However, few if any of those nurses were EMTs! There simply were not many women involved in EMS, in the classroom or in the field. That reality began to change rapidly in the mid-1980s, and*

now I believe that most EMS professionals would agree that women are an integral component of every aspect of emergency services.

Did You Experience Any Gender Discrimination as You Advanced in Your Career?

Deputy Chief Ransom: In the beginning, there was tremendous discrimination unless you stayed on an ambulance. If you thought about being on an engine, there were those who made it clear that you were not wanted and could not do the job. There were a few who believed that women did not belong in any form of EMS or fire and looked at us as a huge burden. Bear in mind, this was not the case with all of the men. There were those who encouraged and supported me to the fullest. It took many years of hard work on the part of most of the women to become accepted and thought of as equals in the department—that is, by those who had no faith in us. With most of the others, all you had to do was show you had a good knowledge of the job and were willing to do any task asked of you.

Ms. Beasley: Most definitely! And my situation was a bit different in that, in our rural area, everyone knew that I was the instructor so they were usually on their best behavior when I was around! But I definitely noticed that females were never first truck unless I pushed the issue, which of course, I did! It was definitely a man's world, and we women were out of place in the eyes of many of the males. The gender discrimination was not directed at me as much as at the other females. Fortunately, I have watched the evolution of that antiquated notion, to the point where we women are accepted and, for the most part, appreciated in our profession. Anyone who doubts that last statement should be on the scene when a new life is entering the world, when a child is injured or gravely ill, when there is a hysterical patient who needs our help, and on and on! At these times, it seems that every male on scene is looking for a female medic! Glean from that what you will.

Do You Think You Practice Leadership Any Differently Than Your Male Counterparts?

Deputy Chief Ransom: After the hardships I faced early in my career, I believe I am more understanding of those who are struggling to do the best job they can (male or female) and offer much encouragement. I also have a tendency to look at things from a mom's perspective, especially with

our younger employees. I am not sure this is the best approach to leadership, but it seems to work for me.

Ms. Beasley: Honestly, I don't tend to look at leadership as gender specific, per se. I think that leadership is, in large part, innate in some individuals and, conversely, a learned behavior in other people. Most assuredly, our leadership styles and abilities vary, based on our willingness to nurture our students, whether they are in-class students or those who, for whatever reasons, have chosen to follow in our footsteps. Covey's roles of modeling and pathfinding really seem to conceptualize my type of leadership. In addition, I have always felt strongly that, if I want to lead any group of individuals, first I have to prove myself worthy of their trust and I have to demonstrate that I will walk beside them right up to the point where we both agree that they are capable of walking on their own.

What Is Your Approach to Practicing Leadership?

Deputy Chief Ransom: I have had several great role models as far as leaders go. Chief Spencer is one of the best role models anyone could have. He is still young, progressive, and well educated. This allows me to see things from another perspective that is up to date. I lead with a hands-on approach as well as by example. I would never expect our personnel to do anything I would not do. Often you find Chief and me out in the middle of an incident working. By this, I mean we are not assuming a command role, but dragging a hose line, rehabbing personnel, or doing any task that needs to be done. When you establish this type of leadership role, your personnel are more apt to work harder by seeing others who do not always have to work on an incident scene doing so.

Ms. Beasley: It is difficult for me to encapsulate my approach to leadership. If I were to take it down to its most basic form, I would simply tell you that I strive to lead by example. I never ask my students or mentorees to do anything that I am not willing to do. And most importantly, I think that I am firm, when need be, and compassionate and understanding when those traits are indicated. And I never confuse the words lead and dictate! To me, it's as simple as this: a leader sets goals, then goes to every conceivable length to meet those goals while explaining the process all along the way. Also, I'm more than willing to learn from those who have been leaders much longer than I have been. It's a delicate balance between being a leader and being a friend/ mentor. I believe that leadership is a learned behavior. In short, I think that a great leader must encompass all of Covey's principles and must be able to walk the walk if they are going to talk the talk!

These two women have obviously done an outstanding job overcoming gender discrimination, rising to the top of their profession and serving as role models to younger women and men coming up through the ranks.

▌ TEAMWORK

What is teamwork? Many people may define teamwork as a group of people working together to accomplish something. Is that really how teamwork is defined? What if each person has a different agenda for participating? Is it teamwork, or just a group of people contributing individually to a project? A team can more meaningfully be defined as follows: "A team is a small group of people with complementary skills who are committed to a common purpose, performance goals, and approach for which they hold themselves mutually accountable" (Katzenbach & Smith, 2003).

Katzenbach and Smith (2003) found a significant difference between teams and working groups. Teams share leadership, the team as an entity and its individuals were accountable for their results, open-ended discussions occurred during meetings that involved problem-solving actions, and team members made decisions together. Work groups were less accountable as a whole. Accountability rested with the individual, but not with the team as a whole. Leadership was given to a single person who had the authority to accept or reject suggestions in the decision-making process. The organization's mission, not the working group, dictated the team's mission.

Chief Jones's greatest challenge is to bring her diverse group of training officers together and get them working as a team to support the new academy's mission. This is not an easy task. In addition to facing resentment from many of her trainers and the gender bias described, Chief Jones must also deal with an organizational culture that typically emphasizes hierarchy over collaboration.

Those in the emergency services professions like to think they work as teams. Yet they are usually directed in their roles by higher-ranking officers and subject to rules, regulations, policies, procedures, and guidelines—all of which inhibit the characteristics of teamwork described

by Katzenbach and Smith (2003). Unlike disaster response, training is an ideal function in which to try to implement genuine teamwork. Using a leadership approach to building her team, Chief Jones could include her senior training officers for each agency in the decision-making process for the training division's roles, objectives, and program development. If she approaches the task with a directive style, she cannot call her group a team. Each person brings her own individual strengths and knowledge to a profession; no individual is the sole expert—not even the chief. Using a team-building approach, one draws on the knowledge, expertise, and experiences of the entire group to produce a better outcome. The leader in this scenario has to work at building trust, allowing input, developing shared leadership, enabling personal and professional growth, and guiding the group to intrinsic and extrinsic motivation.

> ### Leadership Points to Ponder
>
> *A team, on the other hand, is more than the sum of its parts, that is, more than the sum of each person's individual effort.*
>
> Katzenbach and Smith (2003)

Teams take time to develop and gel. One of the most famous development guidelines is Tuckman's sequential stage theory, which states that any group of people go through a definitive developmental process (Tuckman, 1965; Tuckman & Jensen, 1977). The first stage is the forming stage, where members begin to get to know each other, their individual roles, and the rules. The second is the storming stage, where conflict is predominant as members begin to express their ideas, reject ideas, and work through their differences. Third is the norming stage, where agreement is reached on rules, roles, and behavior. During this phase, the team's cohesion increases as members' commitment to the goals increases. The fourth stage is performing, where the actual work occurs. Members solve problems and begin to work efficiently, and real productivity occurs. The fifth and final stage is the adjourning stage. At some point, all teams dissolve or lose members.

Stage two, the storming stage, deserves further attention. Chief Jones has a real challenge here, and how she approaches it is paramount to the success of her training division. She has senior training officers who ran their own training centers for their respective public safety sectors before this merger. Each was the sole person responsible for their agency's training initiatives. Now they are one level down in the hierarchy of the new academy. If Chief Jones chooses to use a coordinator or facilitator approach, this can lead to reduced conflict and smoother transitions. Using an outsider to facilitate lends a degree of nonbias to the decision-making and conflict resolution process. The facilitator needs to be trained to mitigate differences and assist in building this group of individual officers into a team. Each person needs to learn what the others' strengths and weaknesses are and collectively work to enhance their respective divisions. Taking a more directive or passive approach leads to confusion and increased confrontation. The division chiefs are all accountable for their sections and instructors, yet they are also accountable to recruits, personnel, other officers, management, and stakeholders. Working together for a common purpose can lead to better training opportunities and increased comradery between personnel from all agencies.

> A common mistake is to call a work group a team but treat it as a collection of individuals (Hackman, 1990). Teams do not just happen; they are carefully designed and developed. Excellent teams have developed a sense of unity or identification. Such team spirit often can be developed by involving members in all aspects of the process (Larson and LaFasto, 1989). (Northouse , 2007, p.219–220).

As Jones emphasizes collaboration and teamwork, she also needs to make it clear that she will not tolerate infighting and deceit. Training officers who try to highjack the mission or work their own agenda could find themselves relieved of their duties. All leaders have to exercise their authority and make tough decisions from time to time, and Jones is no exception.

Leadership Points to Ponder

When the leader's behavior matches the complexity of the situation, he or she is behaving with "requisite variety," or the set of behaviors necessary to meet the group's needs.

Northouse (2007, p. 209)

CONFLICT MANAGEMENT

Conflict is a normal part of everyday life and a normal function of group interactions (what Tuckman calls the "storming stage"). People have their own perceptions and opinions, even when they do not have a stake in the outcome. Others are wired in such a way that they thrive on controversy. Competition for scarce resources, promotions, policies, and other self-interests are common sources of conflict. According to Dean Tjosvold, past president of the International Association of Conflict Management, conflict can be seen as part of the solution, not as simply an obstacle to progress. People with this outlook, which Tjosvold calls "conflict-positive," encourage healthy conflict and believe that it can be constructive. They also see many values in conflict and recognize how it can create excitement, interest, focus, and a way to solve problems (Tjosvold, 1999).

In the chapter scenario, conflict may arise as training officers from various agencies work together to develop interdisciplinary courses, meet accreditation guidelines, and provide college credit for the academy's new collegiate program, all with no prior working relationships to fall back on for support. When conflict does arise, team members need to approach conflict resolution in a systematic manner, using specific techniques to overcome their differences and arrive at a win-win solution. Next is a list of action items that Chief Jones's staff can draw on to help them navigate and negotiate their differences:

- Acknowledge sources of conflict and dig down to identify the root causes.

- Acknowledge the feelings of others. This is extremely important.

- Present the reason for your opinion and actively listen to the position of others.

- Focus on wants and interests, not just positions, and identify the factual differences between what each side wants. Without understanding what the disagreement is about, there will be no movement to resolution.

- Be flexible. This is a key to successful negotiations.

- Be creative. This can produce innovative ideas and solutions to complex problems, allowing for a mutually agreeable solution.

- Remain motivated to achieve the desired outcome. If parties become unmotivated, find ways to remotivate them. If the conflict continues, the results could be devastating (i.e., lose–lose).

- Keep in mind that with a win–lose approach, there are generally no real winners.

Chief Jones might consider taking a break from the team's training goals to address the issue of conflict management directly and proactively. **TABLE 12-1**, developed by

Table 12-1 Conflict Management—Five Basic Strategies

Owl	Problem-solving negotiations	Values goals and relationships. Solutions are designed to ensure that both parties meet their goals and resolve any tensions.
Teddy Bear	Smoothing	Values relationships more than goals. If your goal is less important than the relationship, you help the other person achieve their goal.
Shark	Forcing or win-lose negotiations	Values goals only; sees no value in the relationship. Forces personal opinions and uses questionable tactics, such as threats, aggression, and penalties to win at all cost.
Fox	Compromising	Moderately values goals and relationships. Realizes that neither can get their way. Will compromise, meeting in the middle, flipping a coin, and so forth, because they do not have time to negotiate.
Turtle	Withdrawing	Values neither the goals nor the relationship. May just walk away with the issue unresolved. May be best in hostile situations until all parties calm down.

Source: Adapted from Conflict Strategy Game. Johnson and Johnson, 2009, p. 375.

Johnson and Johnson (2009), is a great way to get members of her team engaged in a discussion about various constructive approaches to dealing with their differences.

Whatever approach Chief Jones and her staff choose, they need commitment, perseverance, and good faith to succeed. Chief Jones's job is to convince them it is worth the effort and coach them through the process.

BUILDING OUR REPLACEMENTS

Covey (2004) writes about finding the "sweet spot." His Four Roles of Leadership fit neatly into the concept of focus and execution (**TABLE 12-2**). He tells of the influence that Bossidy and Charan (2002) had on his development of *The 8th Habit*. Focus is about dealing with what most matters. Execution is about making it happen. Leaders have the responsibility to lead their followers to that proverbial Promised Land. To accomplish this, they have to do more than give lip service. The old adage "we are going to grow our own" has been around for years, but many people do not know how to accomplish this, or are only speaking hollow words. This statement

means that a person is going to teach you their way of doing things. This occurs in all public safety disciplines from recruit training to promotional processes and even into some higher education institutions. There are national standards, yet a National Professional Qualifications Firefighter or a National Registered Paramedic may not be recognized by a specific state or local jurisdiction and thus have to repeat the same training, or location-specific modules, just to meet these local standards. There is too much variance in what is considered a

Table 12-2 Stephen R. Covey's Four Roles of Leadership

1. Modeling: Inspires trust without expecting it (personal moral authority)
2. Pathfinding: Creates order without demanding it (visionary moral authority)
3. Aligning: Nourishes both vision and empowerment without proclaiming them (institutional moral authority)
4. Empowering: Unleash human potential without externally motivating it (cultural moral authority)

national standard course or certification to be considered such.

Growing our own should not just focus on the local way of doing things; it should be a focus on what is important to one's personnel. How do they achieve personal and professional growth? Focusing on how leaders develop their personnel is an essential part of leadership practice. Does one expect every employee or student to attain perfection? Those who say yes are not being realistic. Each person brings a set of skills and abilities to the table, yet not all will be successful. Where leadership practices enter the equation is when a person provides guidance, opportunities, and every possible resource to personnel to become proficient. Being a servant to these "followers" allows them the best opportunity to succeed. Some will exceed expectations, some will meet them, and others will not. Failure is acceptable when controlled and not done in an environment that can endanger themselves, other responders, or the public. Failing at something can be a great motivator and educational tool, if properly used and not done in a negative or punitive manner. Everyone has failed at something during their lives. Maybe it was a school subject, a project, an idea, or a relationship, but that experience most likely made them stronger and wiser. Leadership is about helping followers adapt and overcome. Each person has a unique opportunity to execute the goal, and to help others succeed.

> ### Leadership Points to Ponder
> Visionary leaders cultivate their followers by being mindful of this one simple thought:
> Teach them to replace you, as someday they will.

Herein lies the question: Will you step up to the plate and take your personnel under your wing, teach them all you know, and encourage them to be better than you? Parents hope their children have things better than they had in their own lives. So why would a person not want the same from those they mentor professionally? Are they not the future of the department? The author challenges the reader to take the lessons learned from this book and apply them to their professional life. Remember the following statement when thinking about one's followers: teach them to replace you, because someday they will—or someday they may have to protect or care for you!

CONCLUSION

Chief Jones has a daunting task ahead. Being the first woman division chief brings with it a unique set of problems, but Chief Jones has demonstrated that she is up to the challenge. Her greatest mountain to climb is managing conflict and building her division into a cohesive group. Team building and conflict management go hand in hand internally as she works to understand each training officer's perspective and power base and overcome whatever resistance she encounters. Externally, she needs to be cognizant that internal strife can affect the dynamics and success of group-to-group negotiations.

Understanding that relationships are key in creating group synergy and high-functioning teams will help Chief Jones execute her strategy. As Rost postulated, leadership is a process of relationship development leading to mutually acceptable outcomes. Jones has the tools, from both job experience and academia, to be successful as a leader by building these relationships. Although Jones carries a high degree of positional authority, acknowledging that she is a servant first goes a long way toward fostering success.

Today's approaches to leadership, and leading, have changed. The industrial paradigm of leadership as power and control is no longer effective in many, if not most, organizations. A paramilitary approach to scene management is still essential in that one person needs to be in charge. Yet on large, catastrophic calls, this is no longer feasible. A multidisciplinary, multiagency response requires influence and savvy to manage. Training and education are keys to developing these skill sets in all responders. The approach that United County is undertaking is one that can lead not only to competent, skilled workers, but to a department where a culture of pride and success prevails.

12

Wrap-Up

ACTIVITY

Using the table below, answer the questions regarding the stakeholders who are beneficial to your agency. Once you have answered each question, identify strategies you will use to build a positive and lasting relationship with each.

Questions	Answer	Strategies to building effective partnership
1. Who are your stakeholders?		
2. Are any stakeholders missing from your list?		
3. What are the key characteristics of positive relationships with stakeholders?		
4. With which stakeholders do you have the most positive relationships right now?		
5. With which stakeholders do you not have positive relationships?		
6. What are your weaknesses in building relationships with each stakeholder?		
7. How can you build trust more effectively?		
8. What strategies do you use to maintain relationships with stakeholders?		
9. What are your strengths and weakness when it comes to political savvy?		

REFERENCES

Bossidy, L., & Charan, R. (2002). *Execution: The discipline of getting things done.* New York, NY: Crown Business.

Covey, S. R. (2004). *The 8th habit: From effectiveness to greatness.* New York, NY: Free Press.

Hulett, D. M., Bendick, M., Thomas, S. Y., & Moccio, F. (2008, April). *A national report card on women in firefighting.* Retrieved from http://www.i-women .org/images/pdf-files/35827WSP

Johnson, D. W., & Johnson, F. P. (2009). *Joining together: Group theory and group skills* (10th ed.). Upper Saddle River, NJ: Pearson.

Katzenbach, J., & Smith, D. (2003). *The wisdom of teams.* Cambridge, MA: Havard Business School Press.

Lips, H. (2009). *Women and leadership: Delicate balancing act.* Retrieved from http://www.womens media.com/lead/88-women-and-leadership-delicate-balancing-act.html

Northouse, P. G. (2007). *Leadership: Theory and practice* (4th ed.). Thousand Oaks, CA: Sage.

Tjosvold, D. (1999). *Conflict management in the asia pacific: assumptions and approaches in diverse cultures.* Hoboken, NJ: John Wiley & Sons.

Tuckman, B. (1965). *Developmental sequence in small groups. Psychological Bulletin,* 63, p 384–399.

Tuckman, B., & Jensen, M. (1977). Stages of small group development revisited. *Group and Organizational Studies,* 2, 419–427.

Index